Shift

A practical guide to
cultivating equity & inclusion
in healthcare education

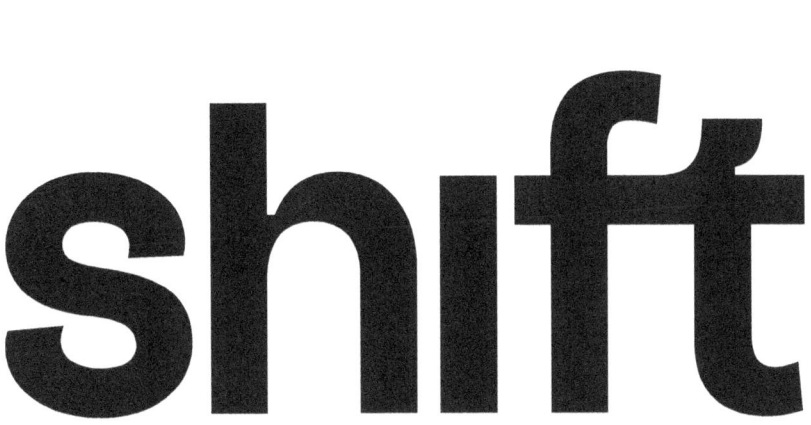

Dr. Sally Arif

EQUITY-
MINDED
COLLECTIVE

Copyright © 2025 by Sally Arif

Published by Equity-Minded Collective, LLC

Cover Design: Nermin Moufti

Figure Design: Shazia Pappa

First Edition

Printed in the United States of America

ISBN: 979-8-9922122-0-4

E-ISBN: 979-8-9922122-1-1

Library of Congress Control Number: 2024927513

www.EquityMindedCollective.com

For inquiries related to permissions and bulk orders, including college textbook/course adoption use please send a message to the publisher at sally@equitymindedcollective.com.

All rights reserved. No part of this publication may be reproduced, distributed, stored in a retrieval system, or transmitted in any form or by any means, electronic, mechanical, photocopying, recording, or otherwise, without prior written permission of the publisher.

Notice

The author and the publisher have made every effort to ensure the accuracy and completeness of the information presented in this book. However, the author and the publisher cannot be held responsible for the continued currency of the information, any inadvertent errors, or the application of this information to practice. Therefore, the author and the publisher shall have no liability to any person or entity with regard to claims, loss, or damage caused or alleged to be caused, directly or indirectly, by the use of the information contained herein. To protect their privacy, the names of some of the people, places, and institutions in this book have been changed.

Dedication

To Yusuf and Yaseen, my forever inspiration.

Table of Contents

Preface 1

Introduction 5

PART I: THE PRELUDE

Chapter 1. How We Got Here 15

Chapter 2. Historical Context and Persisting Barriers 21

Chapter 3. Diversity & Access Laws in Higher Education 31

Chapter 4. The Language and Frameworks of Inclusion 39

Chapter 5. Cycles of Socialization and Narratives 49

PART II: THE PRINCIPLES

Chapter 6. The SHIFT Framework 61

Chapter 7. Self-Reflect Critically 69

Chapter 8. Honor Cultural and Structural Humility 77

Chapter 9. Invite Vulnerability and Discomfort 87

Chapter 10. Foster Connection over Content 97

Chapter 11. Think Active Allyship 105

PART III: THE PRACTICE

Chapter 12. Moving Principles into Action 121

Chapter 13. Intentional Course Design 129

Chapter 14. Equity-Minded Syllabus Development 139

Chapter 15. Equity-Minded Assessments 145

Chapter 16. Facilitation Skills & Intergroup Dialogue 151

Chapter 17. Support Through Restorative Justice 159

Chapter 18. Fostering Affirming Learning Spaces............ 169

Chapter 19. Bias Intervention Techniques 193

Chapter 20. "Cultural Competence" in the Curriculum....... 215

Chapter 21. Health Equity in Experiential Teaching.......... 231

Chapter 22. Case-Based Learning and Simulations 239

Chapter 23. Decolonizing the Curriculum 249

Chapter 24. Sustainability and Metrics for Progress 263

Chapter 25. Continuing Professional Development.......... 273

Chapter 26. Organizational Culture & Inclusive Leadership... 281

APPENDIX

Book Discussion Guide 296

Glossary 299

Notes 305

Acknowledgements 321

Health Equity Pedagogical Resources 323

Preface

"No matter what has happened in our past, when we open our hearts to love we can live as if born again, not forgetting the past but seeing it in a new way. We go forward with the fresh insight that the past can no longer hurt us. Mindful remembering lets us put the broken bits and pieces together again. That is the way healing begins."
—bell hooks

"If you really want to help your patient reach their optimal health, you must first understand them as a person. You must also get curious about how much our society is willing to help them succeed." I stood at the end of a long corridor of the hospital, a final-year pharmacy student on my clinical rotations, wondering how to unpack my preceptor's words. This lesson has stayed with me since.

Growing up as an immigrant and a refugee in a small college town in the heartland of the United States, I (a Turkmeni-Iraqi Muslim girl) realized early on that my personal journey profoundly influenced my unwavering commitment to equity and inclusion in both my personal and professional life. Throughout my childhood, I consistently grappled with feeling like an outsider. In elementary school, I was reluctantly pulled out of my regular classes for daily "English as a Second Language" sessions or ridiculed for having a lunch that was deemed "funny looking" or "smelly" by other kids in the cafeteria.

In middle school, I faced the distressing experience of having my hijab forcefully torn off my head, a brutal message of exclusion

Preface

echoing loudly—"You don't belong here." It wasn't until my college years, particularly in the post-9/11 era, when Islamophobia was heightened, that I truly grasped the complexities of identity and diversity. I leaned heavily into my ability to adapt and connect with others, much like a chameleon—a survival mechanism I initially used to fit in. However, as an adult, this adaptability transformed into an integral part of my healing process, providing me with solace within the tribe of "others" that I had yearned for during my formative years.

It was during my twenties, through meaningful encounters with fellow Muslims and other students socially marginalized, that I finally discovered a profound sense of belonging. Whether it was forming deep friendships with my Korean-American classmates in a predominantly White institution during pharmacy school, finding camaraderie with co-residents who were openly gay during my postgraduate training, or connecting deeply with Muslim and Black colleagues as a professor later in my career, I found sanctuary and understanding in these relationships. I came to realize that the experience of feeling "othered" creates a profound and relatable sense of pain and connection. As you read this, I imagine you may recall similar memories of seeking environments where you could let your guard down and be your authentic self. As humans, we all crave spaces where we don't have to justify our existence or hide out of fear of being misunderstood.

My parents came from humble backgrounds and instilled in me the importance of higher education, continuous learning, and healing. My mother, a pharmacist trained in Iraq, would recount stories of how she and her four sisters were not allowed to marry until they completed their college education. My maternal grandmother, who had only completed the fifth grade, wanted to ensure their success beyond the confines of the home. Similarly, my paternal grandmother, who raised me during my early years before our immigration to the United States, had only completed the seventh grade and went on to have eight children after marrying at a young age. Education was deeply ingrained in my upbringing as a key that unlocked a meaningful and successful life. Curiosity and questioning were at the core of my being and fueled my desire to continuously explore and learn about the diverse world around me.

These experiences and the values instilled in me have shaped my commitment to equity, inclusion, and lifelong learning. They continue to drive me to create spaces where individuals can be seen, heard, and celebrated for their unique identities—fostering a world where diversity is embraced, cherished, and seen as an asset. My past has afforded me a deep exploration of vulnerability, resilience, and the profound impact of exclusion. I have also come to understand and appreciate that integrating diversity, equity, and inclusion (DEI) into education can be deeply complex and nuanced. This is why I have leveraged my nearly two decades of experience in healthcare and higher education to share how I have built effective and integrative work around DEI in often challenging organizational environments. I see the need to achieve equity as a moral necessity in healthcare. As educators, we have a responsibility to model this with our trainees.

My lived experiences have informed me that not everyone is given the resources and opportunities they need, but as a pharmacy student, I had not yet learned what fueled these systems of inequity. Today, after many years of practicing intercultural care and teaching topics related to social justice, health equity, and cultural competence to thousands of healthcare students, I understand that we must practice cultural humility, a lifelong commitment to better understanding each other, and a willingness to interrogate how society assigns value to individuals. I also understand that we are

Preface

never done learning. Putting equity and inclusion into practice is no exception to this rule, regardless of how long we have been in the practice of serving patients or trainees. As long as we are functioning in the current era of our healthcare and education systems, then we are, by default, practicing within inequitable and often non-inclusive environments. If you are an educator, administrator, or healthcare professional who has a desire to contribute to creating inclusive training environments for our students and residents, then I am confident that this book can help you find your path.

Introduction

*"Wherever the art of medicine is loved,
there is also a love of humanity."*
—Hippocrates

I recently attended a lecture on advocacy and justice by Dr. Sherman Jackson, author and professor of Religion, American Studies, and Ethnicity. During his talk, he shared a profound insight that resonated deeply with me: *"We cannot guide people we don't care for."* This reinforced my belief that better learning outcomes for our learners and improved health outcomes for our patients come from prioritizing humanity. Humanity reflects our interconnectedness and involves a recognition of the inherent dignity and worth of every human being. In healthcare education, this means we move away from just algorithmic thinking and embrace the practice of intentional inclusive design infused with empathy and compassion both inside and outside our classrooms. We are not in the business of training biomedical technicians—we are shaping the next generation of healers.

Healthcare providers and educators today must understand the issues that affect the communities they serve and ensure that inclusion and equity is integrated and modeled to our learners. Addressing drivers of health disparities like negative social determinants of health, unconscious bias, anti-racism, and the need to integrate cultural humility into healthcare professional curricula and continuing professional education requirements are essential. This book is not for those who are only looking for data-driven

Introduction

reasons why cultivating inclusive and equitable environments is important to healthcare and education. When we over-intellectualize the provision of care in our healthcare systems and see our patients as mere "capital," this drains us of our inherent humanity. I am past reducing the importance of inclusivity and equity into a mere business case when we cannot overlook that *lives are literally at stake*. There is a moral imperative to doing this work. Like many healthcare professionals and health science educators, no one ever sat me down to give me the insights and steps on how to be an inclusive educator or model how to be an equity advocate. My intention is that this book provides the necessary principles and goalposts to move us forward. I have included examples to help illustrate principles, but full mastery will come through sustained practice over time.

We are here to decenter ourselves and to more authentically center our patients and learners, especially those who carry identities that are rooted in historical socioeconomic disadvantage and under-resourcing. Inclusion work, and ultimately liberation, requires us to not only be brave but also to be truth-tellers. We must be willing to name the tension and not bypass the pain points that make us want to stay comfortable.

To achieve more equitable and inclusive healthcare training programs, a fundamental shift is required.

> A shift to practice humility and honor humanity.
> A shift to an equity-based mindset.
> A shift to inclusive and compassionate pedagogy.
> A shift to center connection over content.
> A shift to restorative practices and respect.

This particular shift involves reimagining the curriculum, dismantling any existing barriers, and embracing a holistic approach that centers on diversity, empathy, and cultural humility. Educators must not only impart knowledge to learners but also

Introduction

do their own critical reflection to foster a mindset of continuous learning and self-awareness. This book takes these concepts from theory to practice as the reader is provided with insights, frameworks, and strategies that can be used to create inclusive and equitable learning environments that support and ensure access and success for all learners, regardless of their identities or backgrounds. By making this transformative shift, we can pave the way for a future where healthcare training programs truly reflect the principles of equity and inclusion and promote a workforce that is prepared to care for a diverse society.

You picked up this book for a reason. What brought you to this book? What is it that you're looking to gain or better understand? Take a moment and write this down. I ask you to revisit your "why" as you explore each chapter. You will find that what initially motivated you to explore the contents of this book may change over time as you engage in learning more about integrating equity, diversity, and inclusion principles into your daily teaching practice and patient care. If we want to advance diversity and inclusion in biomedical sciences and healthcare, we must give our students and residents the individual capacity to ensure health equity. We must empower them as tomorrow's leaders, clinicians, and researchers to contribute to institutional capacity to change the current landscape of health disparities. You may also find that the barriers that keep you from engaging in this work might also shift as you gain knowledge, skills, and understanding. So many people believe that to educate individuals, we need to give them consistent information over and over again. I believe that true learning emerges when individuals feel a part of the experience. My aspiration is that, as you delve into each chapter, you'll recognize yourself in the narrative.

Introduction

Take note of what feelings arise as you read certain chapters. Write those feelings down in the margins and reflect on them. Be mindful of the emotions that arise. Before we can roll up our sleeves and "do the work," we must first understand the principles that guide how the work should be done. Some of the topics covered in this book can feel challenging to explore because they feel overly personal or unfamiliar. Most often, when I am called to provide strategy assistance or educational support to institutions that want to engage in DEI work, they eagerly say, "*We just want the tools and strategies to get the work done.*" While I love the enthusiasm to get to the "how," I am often left worried about the intentions and sustainability of outcomes that are generated without a deep understanding of the "why." Skipping past the thinking and feeling part of this will stifle the authenticity of true progress. For this reason, this book is divided into three sections. Part 1, titled "The Prelude," offers the historical context and insights that have led us to the present moment of observing disparities in healthcare and education. In Part 2, "The Principles," the book presents the theoretical foundations essential for a mindset shift and the profound self-reflection necessary to authentically engage in the work and initiate action. Finally, Part 3, "The Practice," delineates actionable strategies to incorporate DEI concepts into practice, encompassing both educational and real-world settings.

Drawing inspiration from my love of cultural immersion through travel, I envision this book as a preparation for a journey. Before embarking on a trip to a new country, it's advisable to research the destination, learn its language, history, and customs (Part 1), and acquire a guide map for your travels (Part 2). This ensures that you arrive better prepared to maximize your experience and engage thoughtfully with your surroundings (Part 3). Sure, you can just arrive at your final destination without much preparation, but you may not extract the maximum experience—you may even offend the locals by not considering the local customs, traditions, or norms.

Part 3 shifts from an individual-focused exploration of inclusive and equitable learning environments to broader programmatic approaches in later sections. Enjoy the journey, take your time, and feel free to navigate between chapters. Just like revisiting a place, you'll find that ideas resonate differently with each visit, fostering a growing sense of familiarity.

You may be wondering if you are the "right" audience for this book. I intended for this book to assist anyone who may just be starting on the path to creating more inclusive and equitable healthcare learning environments, or even those who have been on the journey for some time. As a guide for pragmatic, outcomes-based strategies for healthcare educators, practitioners, and administrators, this book aims to be both informative and demystifying. This book is not meant to be approached with the intention of boiling the ocean. It is to be used as a guide and reference that should be revisited over and over with the intention of shifting our orientation toward achieving health equity and cultivating a future of culturally sensitive providers.

My perspective as an author is predominantly informed by a US-centric viewpoint, as this is where most of my clinical practice and academic training originates from. While I aim to provide insights that are relevant and valuable across various healthcare education contexts, it is important to acknowledge that my perspective is primarily rooted in the experiences, dynamics, and cultural nuances of an educator and clinician who practices in the United States. In this book, my goal is to share principles, strategies, and frameworks to guide the process of training future healthcare professionals. The ultimate objective is to empower them to analyze

Introduction

systems and instigate the necessary changes to address the root causes of health, social, environmental, and economic inequalities and systems of oppression. The stories I share are true. The names have been changed to honor the confidentiality of those whom I have worked with and taught. When we commit to consistent and measurable DEI initiatives and planning, we not only improve the safety and quality of patient care, including health outcomes, but ensure we retain our talented workforce.

This work does not fall on the shoulders of one individual, group, or community. Inclusivity must be woven into the DNA of healthcare training programs if we want to create a healthier and more equitable future. We each hold a responsibility and privilege to do this work. I intentionally center the movement that is necessary to shift our practices to reach our final destination: humanity in health.

At the time of publishing this book, the term "DEI" and related initiatives have come under significant scrutiny and attack across boardrooms, state legislatures, and college campuses in the United States. That being said, DEI will be the acronym I use to describe the work in this book, and I fully recognize that it is not always used by others. You may have seen words like "accessibility," "belonging," or "justice" integrated into acronyms. These are all important and part of the necessary puzzle pieces, but my goal is not to find the only and best acronym. Rather, it is to engage others in healthcare and education to achieve the goal of equity and justice. I fully expect that, as this book is used, new nomenclature, terminology, and sentiments will emerge in this space. But rather than getting stuck on "the right words," let's not lose sight of the end goal—to serve diverse communities with respect, while upholding the dignity of every individual and honoring our differences.

I will introduce the framework of "SHIFT" in Part 2 of this book because, despite our differences, we all have a collective duty to do better with one another, especially our learners and patients. That's why we are here. With that said, it's important to recognize that your life experiences and values hold significance, shaping the way you engage with this book. As Muhammad Ali aptly put it, "True success is reaching our potential without compromising our values." Pay attention to what resonates with you. Allow the thoughts, emotions, and ideas that surface to marinate, and consider how you can incorporate them into your practice.

I invite you to take the lessons from this book and extend the conversation with your students, residents, colleagues, and the broader community as we collectively work toward cultivating inclusion and equity in healthcare education. To help facilitate these discussions, I've included a discussion guide in the appendix. Whether you're working through these ideas on your own or with a group, I hope the guide sparks thoughtful dialogue and deeper reflection on the book's content.

PART I: THE PRELUDE

"No man can know where he is going unless he knows exactly where he has been and exactly how he arrived at his present place."

—Maya Angelou

CHAPTER 1

•

How We Got Here

"I love America more than any other country in the world, and, exactly for this reason, I insist on the right to criticize her perpetually."
—James Baldwin

Baldwin's quote encapsulates the idea that constructive criticism and critique come from a place of care and concern. When applied to how healthcare is delivered in the United States, this quote suggests that recognizing and openly discussing the inequities present in the healthcare system is not an act of disloyalty but rather demonstrates a genuine concern for the well-being and future of the health of our citizens. It means we acknowledge the flaws, imperfections, and inequalities and embody a sense of social responsibility to make it better. I know it is all a little too heavy. But when educators of our future healthcare professionals integrate diversity, equity, and inclusion principles into their teaching, both in the classroom and in experiential training, they not only elevate a workforce that is empathetic and efficient in healthcare delivery but also spark creative solutions to address the persistent inequalities in our healthcare system. For us to fully understand how we arrived at seeing the disparities that exist in higher education and healthcare, it is crucial to study what led us here in the first place.

There is no doubt that both our healthcare system and institutions of higher learning are experiencing rapid transformation. As a professor and practicing hospital pharmacist, I can attest to the multitude of changes that have occurred over the course of my career and as recently as the COVID-19 pandemic. Similarly, my colleagues in healthcare have also shared their experiences with the ever-increasing demands that are being put on their provision of services as they navigate workload and staffing challenges, new technological integrations, public health emergencies, and regulatory changes, to name just a few. The constant evolution in our field of healthcare requires us to think ahead and reflect on what healthcare will look like in 50 years. At the same time, it also requires us to be innovative and flexible in meeting patient care needs as we strive to advance health equity. Our patient populations are complex and continually diversifying. As healthcare professionals, we must enhance our learners' awareness of how to become culturally sensitive providers and advocates for their patients. The conditions in which healthcare professionals undergo training play a crucial role in establishing lasting solutions to the flawed systems we're tasked with navigating. We must also improve our approaches to providing quality and equitable patient care. Resuming "business as usual" is no longer an option because "business as usual" is simply not working. Applying DEI work to healthcare and education is not based on the feeling of "doing the right thing." I truly wish it was that easy. It is based on historical facts and aims to cultivate a just future. The "why" of integrating cultural humility and content around health equity is based on research and internalization of social and geopolitical factors that set up some to fail and others to succeed "at all costs."

DEI initiatives often center around their benefit to institutions and organizations, whereas their true essence should center around empowering individuals and communities so that new structures can emerge while old ones are dismantled. We must teach and focus on these issues in our curricular plans, teaching delivery, and experiential offerings to our trainees. For instance, I often find there is a palpable but invisible discomfort whenever the history of oppression and anti-Blackness is mentioned in healthcare and higher education settings. We, at the very least, need to name this tension and share the facts that come from our own clinical research. For example, Haider and colleagues' publication on unequal outcomes demonstrated that Black patients who would visit the emergency department fared more poorly after traumatic events compared to their White counterparts. In a more standardized study approach in 1999, Schulman and colleagues showed us that race and sex do influence physicians' decisions to recommend cardiac catheterization to patients presenting with heart attack symptoms, particularly when it comes to Black women. This was backed a few years later, in 2003, by the *Unequal Treatment* report published by the Office of Minority Health, which provided expert evidence of how persons of color experienced discrimination throughout the healthcare system. Over two decades later, these disparities continue to exist today. We should not shield these issues from our students if we expect them to be part of the solution.

In order to empower our students to be change agents, we must develop a comprehensive curriculum that includes diverse perspectives and experiences. One that interweaves the need to be culturally sensitive practitioners who consider the context of historical oppression in our society. To know where we are going, we must first set the stage. This means dedicating time to identify

Chapter 1

the attributes of an educator striving to integrate inclusive practices into their teaching, as well as understanding the barriers to progress.

I believe two foundational principles essential to integrating inclusion and equity in our training programs can be seen as intertwining double helixes as shown in Figure 1: 1) practicing and modeling cultural humility with our learners; and 2) committing to advance health equity.

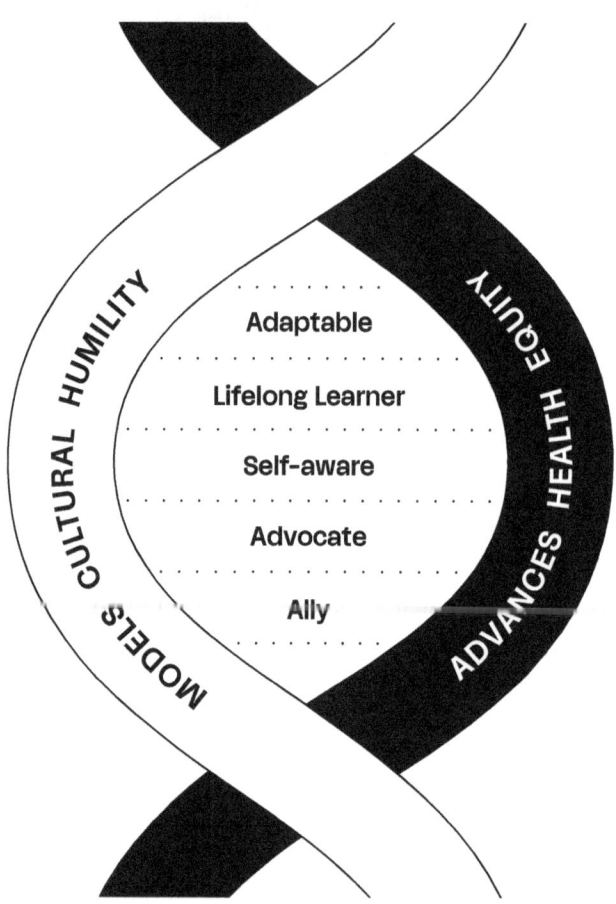

FIGURE 1: ATTRIBUTES OF AN EQUITY-MINDED AND INCLUSIVE EDUCATOR

Regardless of the course we teach or the position we hold within our program, we must recognize the universal individual attributes needed to practice cultural humility and advance health equity within our programs. Ultimately, as healthcare professionals, we must be willing to model our adaptability and life-long learning skills to our learners in the ever-changing landscape of healthcare. We must also be willing to critically self-reflect and gain awareness of our social responsibility to be allies and advocates for our patients and students.

Whether you are just starting in this work or have been mobilizing DEI efforts in your program for some time, I recommend you start by consciously identifying 1) which attributes you are still developing and 2) the solutions needed to overcome any points of resistance in your work. It is natural to feel uncomfortable when engaging in DEI work, but it is just as important to identify active barriers that hinder progress.

Identifying the barriers and possible solutions requires us to practice critical self-reflection. If we aim to build sustainable solutions, we must examine each barrier that is identified within our policies and practices. I've often seen in our contemporary learning environments barriers such as limited administrative or institutional support, inadequate resources like time, money, and space, lack of faculty interest, and professional incentives that are often reported as hurdles to elevating inclusion efforts. *As you read through this book, I ask you to identify any other barriers and possible solutions you might find are present in your own environment.* This allows you to better strategize how to navigate resistance and build capacity to design interventions to teach our students about equitable and inclusive healthcare.

I trust this book will contribute valuable insights to your expanding knowledge, skills, and abilities. We must be willing to commit ourselves to life-long learning and consciously build communities of allies who are willing to disrupt the status quo in order to engage in the process of advocating for our students and patients. From foundational sciences to experiential education, we each hold a responsibility for this work that is ultimately based on celebrating the humanity of care.

Key Takeaways:

1. Understanding the historical and systemic factors that led to current disparities in healthcare and education is crucial for all educators to effectively address and reform these systems.

2. Take responsibility for identifying and addressing the historical systemic barriers in contemporary learning environments and advocate for students and patients by being willing to disrupt the status quo.

3. Two foundational principles for integrating inclusion and equity into in our training programs can be seen as intertwining double helixes (see Figure 1). Both practicing and modeling cultural humility with our learners, as well as committing to advancing health equity, are essential.

CHAPTER 2

•

Historical Context and Persisting Barriers

*"History is not the past, it is the present.
We carry our history with us. We are our history."*
—James Baldwin

I've always found sociological and anthropological perspectives intriguing, especially when exploring identities and discrimination in our broader society and within the healthcare domain. Consider the concept of race, a social construct I first encountered through my upbringing. In our childhood, over the years, my mother consistently reminded me and my brothers that we were not White. Since there was no context for being "White" in our home country of Iraq, it was difficult to understand. In Iraq, identity was often drawn across religious or ethnic lines. Years later, as an educator, I was often assumed to be White because of my easily pronounceable first name, less melanated skin and outward appearance. As a healthcare professional, I routinely observed that the topic of race turned into an academic discussion about healthcare disparities and the need for cultural competency training to navigate our differences better. However, these discussions often overlooked a crucial aspect—the issue of racial and ethnic disparities in healthcare wasn't solely an academic or contemporary research question; it was deeply rooted in a history of oppressive practices.

I attended a health equity conference hosted by Harvard Medical School, where I heard speaker Sherita Golden, Vice President and Chief Diversity Officer for Johns Hopkins Medicine, say, "Our past informs our future." I remember immediately agreeing with this statement but also thinking to myself, doesn't the past also inform our present? Shouldn't we start by looking at what is going on around us first? It is important to understand how we got to the "here" and "now." Current healthcare practice continues to be filled with many of the same health disparities we have seen play out for decades. We must understand that the current path we are traveling along is riddled with remnants of the past. To truly understand the present and the future, we must be well-versed in what has happened in the past.

Learning from historical mistakes is crucial to preventing their repetition. By studying past instances of healthcare discrimination, students can actively contribute to breaking the cycle of inequities and ensuring that such injustices are not perpetuated in the future. For example, the historical discrimination and racism that occurred during slavery and the post-Civil War era should be studied and integrated into our health profession training programs. Understanding the impact of these events on the marginalization of patients and the role of racial categorization in shaping oppressive and exploitative practices in science and medicine is critical to realizing how we got here. The reality is that the historical context of inequities is often never considered or sidelined in our curricula and programming. As a result, an average health science student lacks awareness of the impact of these events on present-day healthcare delivery. Sharing historical examples of healthcare discrimination and racism with our trainees can help equip them with the awareness, empathy, and knowledge needed to contribute to a more equitable and just healthcare system. Here are just a few examples centered around race and ethnicity that can be integrated into our teaching:

- Eugenics theory that defined certain races and ethnicities as biologically inferior to others, including Black and Jewish immigrants.

- Injustices of Dr. J Marion Sims, who went on to be the president of the American Medical Association, despite performing gynecological experiments involving vesicovaginal fistulae procedures on 12 enslaved women from 1844 to 1849. These experiments were without anesthesia nor consent, under the precedent that Black people didn't feel pain the same way as non-Black individuals did. What's even more shocking is that 40% of first- and second-year medical students surveyed endorsed the belief that "Black people's skin is thicker than white people's."

- The Homestead Act of 1862 led to further encroachment on Indigenous lands and displacement of Native American populations. This displacement often resulted in the disruption of traditional health practices and access to resources that were essential for the health and well-being of Indigenous communities.

- In 1910, the U.S. Public Health Service & Bureau of Immigration built a facility to "sanitize" Mexican and other Latino/a/x immigrants, which eventually resulted in the court case of Madrigal v. Quilligan in 1975. So, we shouldn't be surprised when we learn that 1 in 5 Hispanic people report they avoid medical care because of concerns that they will be treated poorly or will be discriminated against again.

- In the educational realm, the closure of medical schools training Black physicians in the 1910s and the lack of Black, Indigenous, and other underrepresented students of color in the biomedical training programs carried forth since.

- Historical relevance of experimentation that occurred on vulnerable groups without their consent with the infamous Tuskegee Study that started in 1932, and impacted clinical trial design and research for decades to come.

This is also layered on the fact that often, our trainees, if given the space to share their experiences, can add to this list of well-known historical events with their own personal accounts of an oppressive healthcare system. A first-generation Black student in one of my public health courses shared the following: *"For a long time, I've been aware that racism plays a large part in why certain populations are treated differently within the healthcare space and other sectors of society. As a [Black] woman myself and having racist experiences within the healthcare space, it is part of why I wanted to enter into a career in healthcare. My most memorable experience was the first time I ever got blood drawn. The phlebotomy tech, who was White, used the needle to feel around inside my arm for a vein and then said, 'You all have such difficult veins,' as the reason she couldn't hit the vein (even though she did not feel around much prior to inserting the needle). I didn't realize this was how this shouldn't be done until I went and got blood drawn a second time, and the tech had a smoother procedure and hit the vein in that same arm on the first try. For the first tech, I had barely moved and tried to be as still as possible while she was (what I believe was intentional) inflicting pain upon me. I knew it wasn't right at that moment and had immediately reported her, but I didn't realize the other steps she was supposed to take to keep me safe until I went for the second blood draw. As a future healthcare professional, I always want to be an advocate and an available source of information for minority patients who want to have more input and information on their care and also be someone who is a listening ear that will also be vocal about any issues they encounter to ensure change."*

> *"Of all the forms of inequality, injustice in healthcare is the most shocking and inhumane."*
> —Martin Luther King Jr.

Our trainees should also understand that healthcare discrimination is often considered a microcosm of broader societal discrimination. This means that the biases, inequalities, and systemic issues that exist in society at large are reflected and sometimes amplified within the healthcare system. As educators, we need to be more transparent with our learners so they better understand the interconnectedness of healthcare discrimination and societal discrimination. For instance, the practice of redlining and predatory lending, which began in numerous US cities in the 1930s, resulted in structural inequalities, racial segregation, and housing insecurity for Black communities. Consequently, these communities continue to face ongoing challenges such as limited access to quality healthcare, reduced patient-provider engagement in decision-making, and lower health literacy levels. This has led to the social determinants of health domains we are all familiar with, as where people live, grow up, learn, worship, and work dramatically impacts their health outcomes. I still remember being surprised to read in the Boston Globe that the median net worth of a White family was $247,500, while the median net worth of a non-immigrant Black family was just $8 in 2017. The economic instability across racial lines I know

Chapter 2

as a clinician translates to compromised health and well-being for my patients. Unfortunately, what is more alarming is that so many hospital leaders and clinicians do not believe that disparities exist when delivering healthcare to different populations. We must start by examining the evidence to provide quality and equitable care. Beyond the fact that health equity is a moral and practical imperative, we also have to focus on the evolving metrics necessary to prove this.

Into the Metrics

In healthcare, we often like to admire problems and diagnose them with limited data. I think it is more important that we be willing to roll up our sleeves and face the messy, uncomfortable past if we really want to find remedies for our current problems. Often, the struggle for most clinicians who witness health disparities among vulnerable populations is the shortfall of policies and practices in healthcare because our metrics have been missing. Metrics help inform change, and we need our trainees to be aware of health equity metrics that help integrate the social needs of patients in our practice settings. As of 2023, various external hospital and health equity metrics have been developed as part of regulatory requirements to help stratify quality, safety, and clinical outcomes across racial and ethnic lines. When it comes to reporting metrics, we might find different standards across organizations. For example, The Joint Commission (JC) is requesting an assessment of health-related social needs and the provision of referral resources. The Centers for Medicare and Medicaid Services (CMS) is requesting the percentage of patients screened for and identified as having food insecurity, housing instability, transportation problems, utility difficulties, and interpersonal safety concerns across all disparities we see in our systems. While this is a more stick-reactive approach to rectifying injustices in healthcare, ultimately, our teaching should stress that regulatory agencies like the Joint Commission and CMS are holding healthcare systems accountable to recognize the drivers of healthcare disparities, develop written action plans, and have data inform how patients across racial and ethnicity lines experience disparities in quality and safety.

It is important to instill in our trainees the need to record social determinants of health (SDOH) data across the health system, and we must do so by utilizing a patient-centered care model. For example, Johns Hopkins uses a patient-centered care model that operates through principles like:

- Routinely incorporating social risk data into care decisions.
- Designing and implementing integrated care systems using approaches that engage patients, community partners, frontline staff, social workers, care managers, community health workers, and clinicians in planning and evaluation.

Data-driven interventions use evidence and research to identify disparities, measure progress, and tailor interventions for specific populations. Collecting and analyzing data helps inform decision-making and evaluate the effectiveness of our interventions. For example, hospitals and healthcare organizations that aim to comply with the National Culturally and Linguistically Appropriate Services (CLAS) Standards are responsible for implementing a range of metrics and indicators to ensure that they are providing equitable and culturally sensitive care. The National CLAS Standards are a set of guidelines and practices developed by the U.S. Department of Health and Human Services Office of Minority Health to ensure that healthcare organizations provide equitable and culturally sensitive care to all patients, regardless of their cultural or linguistic background. The National CLAS Standards function around the principal standard that we must provide effective, equitable, understandable, and respectful quality care and services that are responsive to diverse cultural health beliefs and practices, preferred languages, health literacy, and other communication needs. This includes how we communicate and provide language assistance, especially to individuals who have limited English proficiency.

The key question is how can we encourage our students and residents to engage more deliberately with the historical context and current standards for health equity? There isn't a singular history lesson or planned intervention that can achieve this comprehensively. Instead, we should recognize the various avenues available to spotlight these concepts for our students. One effective method is through the use of case studies. For instance, I often use the White-Black racial gap in life expectancy and the disparities observed in hypertension rates, which are highest among non-Hispanic Black males. Within this disparity, we can investigate the impact of SDOH, team-based care strategies that strengthen community and clinical collaboration, and the appropriate use of race-conscious medicine. In my discussions with my learners, I emphasize the importance of meeting patients where they are and bringing their stories into our treatment plans. I have done this by teaching my students about the infamous hypertension barbershop study published in the *New England Journal of Medicine* in 2018. It highlighted an intervention that Black-owned barbershops were a safe space where Black-American men were treated with respect and trust. It also highlighted a team approach that included a physician-pharmacist collaboration that was embedded into the community to improve lifestyle and medication adherence and resolve social barriers in the health centers we use.

In recent years, we have gained a higher level of consciousness about health disparities that have existed for years, if not decades. Now, it's time to shift our mindset and practices to actively dismantle the systems that perpetuate these inequities. We need to move beyond superficial gestures and commit to meaningful action. This requires understanding the historical context of these disparities and employing data-driven approaches to develop effective solutions. We must show our trainees that achieving equitable health outcomes for their patients depends on their involvement in transforming the healthcare system.

Key Takeaways:

1. To address current health disparities, it is crucial to study the historical discrimination and racism in healthcare, including past experimentation and unequal treatment based on race, ethnicity, and other historically marginalized identities.

2. Healthcare organizations must be aware of health equity metrics and integrate social determinants of health (SDOH) data when operationalizing patient-centered care models.

3. Achieving health equity requires a long-term vision and a commitment to teaching our learners that we must dismantle and rebuild the systems perpetuating inequities.

CHAPTER 3

•

Diversity & Access Laws in Higher Education

"Our work is not done. Each generation must do its part to bring us closer to true freedom and justice."
—John Lewis

Research shows that diversifying our campuses benefits all students, embodying the aphorism, "a rising tide lifts all boats." Beyond just having a diverse student body, education equity ensures that every learner has equal access to a high-quality education and a safe, supportive learning environment. In order to respect this concept in our contemporary times, we must also recognize the consequences of discrimination in our settings of higher learning and clinical care. Discrimination in higher education and medical training has been shown to affect the mental and emotional well-being of learners, leading to higher rates of anxiety, depression, sadness, helplessness, and low self-esteem. We also see effects on cognitive health, with research demonstrating that when students experience daily discrimination, their memory can decline dramatically. Discrimination also impacts physical health, increasing the risk of cardiovascular disease, diabetes, and respiratory diseases like asthma. Individuals who experience daily discrimination also report sleep disturbances and daytime fatigue.

Numerous benefits come with diversifying our trainees and educators within our program.

- **Innovation:** When our student body is diverse, we see 1.7 times more likelihood of producing innovative leaders in healthcare fields.
- **Creativity:** Each identity brings with it different perspectives, which not only increases problem- solving but also creativity when brainstorming ideas.
- **Efficiency:** The more diverse our teams are, the faster we will be able to solve problems, according to a Harvard Business Review study.
- **Engagement:** When there is a culture of inclusion and diversity there is a higher rate of engagement and retention.
- **Improved health:** U. S. Department of Health and Human Services (HHS) Office of Minority Health notes that undeserved populations get better access to high quality care when there is racial or ethnic concordance between patient and provider.

I am not the most enthusiastic student of history, but as I grew in my DEI work, I realized the importance of understanding the historical context of educational laws. The knowledge gained has helped me better understand the societal, political, and cultural factors that shape our educational policies and practices in higher education. On a practical level, immersing myself in our history has provided me with valuable insights for making informed decisions in various aspects of my role, including instructional strategies, my stance on admissions criteria, curricular design, and even classroom management. Specifically, there have been several laws and court cases that have changed the diversity landscape and addressed discrimination in higher education in the United States over the past century. These laws and court cases have played an important role in promoting equal access to educational opportunities for all individuals. However, by no means does this imply that adequate representation of diversity within the health professions has been achieved.

Laws:

- **The Second Morrill Act of 1890:** A federal law that provided funding for the establishment of Historically Black Colleges and Universities (HBCUs) in the United States. The law required states to provide land-grant colleges and universities for African American students in addition to those already established for White students under the original Morrill Act of 1862. This law helped to promote diversity in higher education by providing access to higher education for African Americans who were previously excluded from many universities and colleges. The HBCUs established under the Second Morrill Act of 1890 have played a significant role in providing educational opportunities for African American students and have produced many notable alumni who have made important contributions to society in various fields, including politics, the arts, and science. Today, HBCUs continue to serve as important centers of higher education for students of all backgrounds, promoting diversity and inclusion in higher education.

- **Civil Rights Act of 1964:** This legislation prohibited discrimination on the basis of race, color, religion, sex, or national origin in any program or activity receiving federal financial assistance. This had a significant impact on higher education, as many universities receive federal funding. Furthermore, Title IX of the Education Amendments of 1972 banned sex discrimination. Many people often think of collegiate sports when Title IX bans sex discrimination in programs traditionally dominated by one gender, which can occur in STEM education. Beyond protecting victims of sexual harassment and assault, it also prohibits higher education institutions from denying admission to pregnant applicants or student parents.

- **The Higher Education Act (HEA) of 1965:** A federal law that aims to support and improve higher education in the United States. It established programs and policies to increase access to higher education, improve the quality of education, and provide financial assistance to students. The HEA created a framework for federal student aid programs, including grants, loans, and work-study programs, and established the Free Application for Federal Student Aid (FAFSA). It also created the National Teacher Corps to recruit and train teachers in high-need areas and provided funding for research and development in higher education. Over the years, the HEA has been amended and expanded to address emerging issues and challenges in higher education, such as establishing the Federal Pell Grant program in 1972, which is considered a cornerstone for African American higher education. From 2015 to 2016, more than 50% of Black undergraduate students received Pell grants. Federal student loans, the TRIO program, and the work-study program were also created under HEA.

- **The Rehabilitation Act of 1973:** A law that banned discrimination against people with disabilities. Section 504 of the act provided further protection to federally funded colleges in which any applicants with disabilities could not be treated differently. As universities, both public and private, typically receive federal funds via grants and contracts, they are obligated to adhere to legislative mandates from this ACT as well as the 1990 Americans with Disabilities Act (ADA), which includes Title II, where individuals with disabilities should not be denied the benefit of participating in public entities like colleges and universities.

- **Affirmative Action:** During the civil rights movement and as late as the 1970s, more than 80% of undergraduates were White. Affirmative action has created more diversification in the student landscape by increasing representation through policies and practices designed to promote diversity and increase opportunities for historically underrepresented groups, such as racial and ethnic minorities, women, and individuals from low-income backgrounds. Affirmative action in higher education often involves the consideration of race or ethnicity as a factor in admissions decisions, along with other factors such as academic achievement, extracurricular activities, and socioeconomic status. Proponents of affirmative action argue that it helps to redress past and current discrimination and promotes equal opportunity. Critics argue that affirmative action is unfair to other students and may result in "reverse discrimination." Affirmative action policies have been the subject of several court cases, including the landmark Supreme Court cases of Regents of the University of California v. Bakke (1978), Grutter v. Bollinger (2003), and Fisher v. University of Texas at Austin (2016). Most recently, in

Chapter 3

2023, the Supreme Court of the United States (SCOTUS) upheld an affirmative action ban, ruling that states have the authority to prohibit the consideration of race or ethnicity in college admissions. The ban could lead to a decrease in the enrollment of underrepresented minority students in healthcare professional schools, sending a message that the pursuit of diversity and equity in education is devalued and diminishing the progress made in creating diverse and inclusive higher education environments, forcing institutions to explore new strategies to ensure equitable access for underrepresented students.

Court Cases:

- **Brown v. Board of Education (1954):** This landmark Supreme Court case declared that segregation in public schools was unconstitutional. This paved the way for increased diversity at all levels of education, including higher education. However, it wasn't until 1964 that the Civil Rights Act was passed to end legal segregation.

- **Regents of the University of California v. Bakke (1978):** This Supreme Court case ruled that universities could consider race as a factor in admissions but not as the sole determining factor.

- **Gratz v. Bollinger (2003) and Grutter v. Bollinger (2003):** These two Supreme Court cases upheld the use of race as a factor in admissions decisions but also established that strict quotas or point systems based solely on race were unconstitutional.

- **Fisher v. University of Texas at Austin (2016):** This Supreme Court case reaffirmed the use of race in admissions decisions but also emphasized the importance of a "holistic" approach that considers multiple factors, including race, in order to achieve diversity.

Understanding the laws and cases that shaped equitable education promotes awareness of the ongoing struggle for equality, the importance of maintaining vigilance against discrimination across our campuses, and the impact it can have on diversifying our healthcare workforce. This awareness helps create an even broader society that values diversity and inclusion. While many of these court cases and laws were essential to diversifying higher education and reducing discrimination, they did not provide specific methods for higher education institutions to create programs to support historically excluded groups. For example, within the first two years of college, students with disabilities face not only discrimination based on ableism but also a lack of accessibility to educational technology or physical accommodations, leading to a 35% dropout rate. As educators, we must be well versed not only in the historical context of discrimination and laws that have paved the way for more equity but also understand the language of DEI to move forward. Navigating these laws should come with application to our current landscape for our learners who carry historically marginalized identities.

The goal of diversifying the healthcare profession workforce is important. With 19% of registered nurses being of color in 2022, the American Association of Colleges of Nursing (AACN) stated that one of their top priorities was to diversify the nursing workforce in order to achieve health equity and improve patient care, satisfaction, and adherence. Countless studies have shown how powerful racially concordant provider-patient relationships are to the provision of equitable and culturally competent care. This need for diversity is also seen across other health profession programs.

Chapter 3

In the same breath that we discuss the need to expand and support a diverse future healthcare workforce, we must also recognize how trauma from life experiences associated with a marginalized status can hold back students from pursuing a career in healthcare. For students who have been economically or socially disadvantaged, there are often fewer clear pathways to leadership, limited financial resources, and a lack of mentorship, sponsorship, and overall support to get into postgraduate programs or advance their learning opportunities. We must actively work to remove these barriers and create an inclusive environment that fosters the success of learners who historically have faced systemic and structural exclusion.

Key Takeaways:

1. Discrimination in higher education and medical training adversely affects the mental, emotional, cognitive, and physical well-being of learners, highlighting the importance of addressing equity in healthcare education.

2. Diversifying our healthcare training programs leads to increased innovation, creativity, efficiency, engagement, and improved equitable health outcomes for patients.

3. Understanding the historical context and legal frameworks, including laws such as the Second Morrill Act, the Civil Rights Act, and Affirmative Action, allows educators to navigate and address inclusion in healthcare education more effectively.

CHAPTER 4

•

The Language and Frameworks of Inclusion

"Language is power, in ways more literal than most people think. When we speak, we exercise the power of language to transform reality. Why don't more of us realize the connection between language and power?" —Julia Penelope

The goal of inclusive practices and policies is to cultivate a sense of belonging, whether that is for our students, patients, or colleagues in healthcare. While it can be liberating to share our authentic selves without shame in a group, it can also be frightening when we are asked to express ourselves in an unsafe and unwelcoming environment. Just the mere thought of being the "only" in a classroom or on a team can stifle a person's abilities to grow, learn, and achieve. Words like "isolated," "disengaged," and "anxious" are just some of the common responses I receive when I ask participants in my workshops to respond to the prompt: *"Think of a time you didn't belong to a group. How did it make you feel?"* It often doesn't matter what identity a person holds; there is a universal desire to be accepted and included. Why would our students or trainees feel any different? And why is it often so challenging for us to hold space for students to express themselves authentically in our programs? In Maslow's hierarchy of needs, the sense of belonging holds the third position in significance, preceded only by basic physiological needs and safety. For graduate students, this requirement includes the need for academic belonging, students' social support, and connections within the broader campus community. Belonging doesn't mean just "fitting in," where we bend ourselves to assimilate into the larger group; it's about being genuinely welcomed and respected for who we are. You can't tell someone they belong. They can only determine that based on the choices of inclusion made for them in their environment.

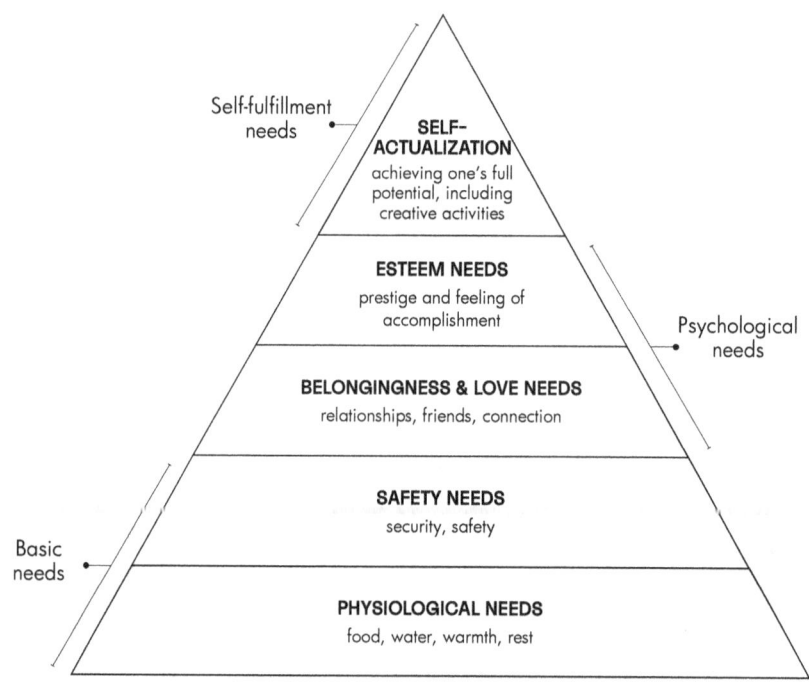

FIGURE 2: MASLOW'S HIERARCHY OF NEEDS

Watch Your Language!

Author Alice Walker put it best when she said, *"Healing starts where the wound is,"* and we can't shift to healing our problems unless we first recognize the historical wounds. This requires us to use shared language to engage in meaningful dialogue that will heal the inequities in higher education and healthcare we have reviewed in the previous chapters. Through the countless DEI workshops I have facilitated for students and healthcare professionals, I have found that we are not only at different places in our journeys, but often, we are not even speaking the same language. Many buzzwords and terms associated with DEI are often tossed around, leading to confusion or misuse. I also find that the ever-evolving DEI lexicon can feel daunting, and is a very common reason why many educators push pause when it comes to engaging in the work. Educators may struggle to keep up with the latest terminology and best practices with inclusive language. Here's the bottom line about DEI-related language: it is not static, and I can safely assume that by the time you are reading this book, some of the language I use will be outdated. This means we must embrace the ongoing commitment to learning and adapting to new terminology.

As educators, we may encounter resistance from students and colleagues when promoting inclusive language if it is perceived as excessive political correctness or "woke" liberal semantics. Some individuals might view using inclusive language as an additional task or inconvenience, especially if they are not personally impacted by exclusionary language. Using inclusive language is not about policing, censorship, or forcing individuals to use only specific words; it's about inviting folks to think about the impact of their words. Individuals may unintentionally use biased language due to societal conditioning and implicit biases, which can perpetuate stereotypes and exclude certain groups. Unless we all get on the same page about the words we use, we cannot solve problems and integrate solutions toward building inclusive and equitable campuses or healthcare institutions. Fulfilling our individual and collective responsibility to DEI means using inclusive language, which can come in various forms:

- **Use gender-inclusive language:** Avoid assumptions about gender. Use gender-neutral terms like "they/them" pronouns when referring to an individual whose gender is unknown. Also, use "students" or "colleagues" instead of gendered terms like "guys" or "ladies."
- **Respect pronouns:** Always use individuals' pronouns. When introducing yourself or asking others for pronouns, normalize the practice to create a safe space for everyone.
- **Avoid stereotypes:** Refrain from using stereotypes or making assumptions about cultures, races, genders, abilities, or other identities. Treat individuals as unique and diverse.
- **Be mindful of cultural sensitivity:** When discussing cultural topics, ensure that your language is respectful and free from stereotypes or biases. Acknowledge that there is diversity within the same cultural group.
- **Address students by their chosen name:** If a student uses a different name from their legal name or one provided by the registrar's office, make an effort to use the chosen name consistently in class and on course materials. You can also utilize pronunciation guides to help avoid mispronunciations and show respect for linguistic diversity.
- **Include diverse representation in your content:** Choose examples, case studies, and scenarios that are inclusive of diverse identities and experiences. This helps all students relate to the content.
- **Provide content or disclaimer warnings:** If course materials contain potentially triggering or sensitive content,

provide content warnings to give students the opportunity to prepare emotionally.

- **Facilitate open discussions:** Create an environment where students feel comfortable expressing their opinions and experiences. Encourage respectful dialogue and ensure that everyone's perspective is valued.

- **Use inclusive language in assessments:** When designing assignments and assessments, ensure that the language used is accessible and does not inadvertently favor one group over another. Avoid colloquial examples in your patient cases or scenarios that are ambiguous or open to interpretation. For example "a meal that didn't sit well" could be revised to "abdominal pain following a meal."

Starting at the beginning means we define important key terms to gain clarity about their meaning and address the nuances. While diversity is the representation of different social or personal groups, inclusion is the intentional choice we make to ensure that individuals who carry various identities can authentically participate in our organizations. I often think of the analogy inclusion strategist and thought-leader Verna Myers makes: *"Diversity is being invited to the party. Inclusion is being asked to dance."* When we build a shared understanding of the language, we use the same dictionary of definitions that helps us move collectively forward together.

- **Diversity:** The wide variety of shared and different personal and group characteristics among human beings that is seen as a representation, often across social identity lines (e.g., race, gender, age, ability, etc.).

- **Equity:** The fair treatment, access, resources, and opportunities for all people. Equity considers social

Chapter 4

> identifiers (i.e., race, socioeconomic status, etc.) faced with inequalities needing to be overcome.

- **Inclusion**: Creating environments through action that authentically bring traditionally excluded individuals and/or groups into the group through a welcoming, supported, and valued environment where they can fully participate and grow.
- **Belonging**: A sentiment or feeling of being connected and accepted in which a person can thrive, reinforced by the organization's culture.

Unpacking Key Terms

As we learn about new terms, we should take time to digest their meaning, unpack, and reflect on what they mean to us. Let's tease out words like equality versus equity. When we say "equality," we should think about sameness. Every student receives the same materials, resources, and opportunities. Every clinician would get the same size lab coat. We should recognize that this approach assumes everyone begins at the same starting point, has the same needs to succeed, and follows a "one size fits all" model. In education, equality is often the easier approach because it requires less effort upfront to acknowledge our audience's differences and to be transparent about our methods and practices. When we think of "equity," we tailor the distribution of resources and opportunities through the lens of difference and its roots to a framework of justice. This can be challenging because it requires the educator to engage in a more personalized and student-centered approach, which can be more time-intensive than an equality-based pedagogical approach. Unpacking equity, we can recognize that historically, systems have included both advantaged and disadvantaged groups. In education, this means that some students do not have the same privileges afforded to them as they navigate the higher education landscape. Filtering our processes and policies through a truly "fair" approach means we set our academic goals for our students through an equity-minded lens. Equity ultimately gives us a better approach when addressing the unique needs and challenges of all students, especially those from historically marginalized or disadvantaged backgrounds. An equity approach ensures that every student has an equal opportunity to prosper in their education journey and requires a proactive evaluation of the unique needs of its students when it provides resources to address their needs. For example:

- Students with disabilities receive accessible formats of textbooks and digital resources.
- Students from low-income backgrounds are offered financial assistance to purchase required materials.
- Multilingual learners are provided with additional language support resources.

As educators, we must also recognize that there are divisive concepts in legislation affecting higher education that have already created inequitable learning environments (see Chapter 3). As institutions of higher learning, we must also invest time in surveying how this leads to exclusion and lack of belonging. Utilizing vetted tools, such as the Persistence in the Sciences (PITS) survey and the Psychological Sense of School Membership (PSSM) Scale, can help us assess the sense of belonging in the sciences. Simply integrating a Likert-based question into an end-of-course evaluation asking, "Did the instructor create an environment that was inclusive or promote a sense of belonging in class?" can help students see that their feeling of belonging is essential to course delivery and design.

The Center for Urban Education (CUE) defines equity-mindedness as "the perspective or mode of thinking exhibited by

Chapter 4

practitioners who call attention to patterns of inequity in student outcomes. These practitioners are willing to take personal and institutional responsibility for the success of their students and critically reassess their own practices. It also requires that practitioners are race-conscious and aware of the social and historical context of exclusionary practices in American Higher Education." This requires the educator to understand that equity is grounded in both equal access and outcomes. It also requires the educator to be conscious of policies, practices, and structures that promote or sustain inequities throughout the institution.

Here's the tricky and often difficult part of employing an equity-minded approach: As educators, we must recognize that our learners are currently operating in a world that is built to advantage some and disadvantage others. While we simultaneously try to build fairness into our practices, we are also trying not to perpetuate further harms on those who are most marginalized historically. It is like putting out a fire in a house from the inside. Many healthcare educators may also lack the training and professional development necessary to implement equity-minded teaching strategies, which can hinder effective progress. Additionally, higher education systems and practices often have a long history of being resistant to change with a "this is how we've always done it" mindset. You might be wondering, "Where do I start as an individual?" Challenging the status quo can start with familiarizing yourself with commonly used equity-minded frameworks. This book will guide you through a few key examples, including:

- **Culturally Responsive Teaching:** focuses on integrating cultural competence into the curriculum, teaching methods, and interactions with learners. This theory aims to acknowledge and respect the diverse cultural backgrounds and perspectives of learners and patients, ensuring that education is relevant and effective for all.

- **Universal Design for Learning (UDL):** aims to accommodate diverse learning styles, abilities, and backgrounds. UDL involves providing multiple means of representation, engagement, and expression in the curriculum to ensure that all students can access and engage with the material.

- **Trauma-Informed Education:** acknowledges that some students may have experienced trauma, which can impact their learning and well-being. Trauma-informed education involves creating a safe and supportive learning environment, being sensitive to triggers, and offering resources for mental health and support.

Key Takeaways:

1. The aim of cultivating inclusion and equity is to foster a sense of belonging, leading to healing and progress.

2. Establishing a shared language and definitions is crucial to effectively address inclusion challenges in healthcare and education and requires a focus on counternarratives that better allow for the tailored distribution of resources, acknowledging historical disadvantages, and promoting justice for excluded groups.

3. Equity-mindedness involves recognizing patterns of inequity, taking responsibility for student success, and being conscious of the historical context of exclusionary practices.

CHAPTER 5

•

Cycles of Socialization and Narratives

"Education is the key to unlocking the world, a passport to freedom. In a world divided by ignorance and intolerance, it is our responsibility to lift our own burdens and reach out to those who suffer."

—Oscar Arias Sánchez

Learners who carry a label of being "underrepresented" or "minority" in the field of STEM are often persons with disabilities, women, Black or African American, Latino or Hispanic, and American Indians or Alaska Natives. These labels are used because these individuals have not been represented and, therefore, don't see their viewpoints or stories represented in STEM disciplines early on in their undergraduate degrees. This omission is loud and speaks volumes about contemporary practice in higher education. To add insult to injury, the default lens often used in higher education STEM programs is that of a cisgendered, straight, White, Christian, and male. This "dominant lens" shapes many of the narratives that are secured as "the right or correct way" or "standard" when health sciences are taught. Pause for a moment and process how this makes you feel. Tense? Angry? Unfazed? It is critical for educators to understand this and explore how to shift the collective narrative to be more inclusive in our learning spaces.

According to the Center for Research on Learning and Teaching (CRLT) at the University of Michigan, minoritized students report that the climate (anxiety levels, how welcome they feel by instructors, etc.) in which they learn heavily influences their decision to stay in STEM disciplines, including healthcare. When students choose to leave our programs, it is a good sign that we need to investigate our narratives and interrogate what lens we are operating from in our instruction and mentoring. This becomes even more critical if we have a programmatic goal to recruit underrepresented graduate students.

"Othering" causes anyone to become self-conscious and disengaged. It says, "You are not part of the team and a burden to the collective." Feeling isolated because you are the "only one" or one of the few can make you feel like an imposter in the workplace. Feelings of self-doubt can stem from not feeling like others believe in you. The entire learning environment is riddled with subtle, problematic messages and behaviors that promote "othering." We have to center inclusivity and access in our learning environments if we expect all of our learners to be successful. Feelings of anxiety and stress grow when a student with limited vision can't see your PowerPoint presentation or a learner is unable to observe designated religious prayer times due to a back-to-back class schedule. These feelings impede the learning process and are primed to occur when accommodations are an oversight by the instructor or program. Providing tools and resources, including time and space, to allow students to meet their academic potential is essential to creating equitable learning environments.

Examining Narratives

I remember the first time I learned about dominant and counter-narratives. After this, I could never unsee all the dominant narratives around me and my environment—in the media, in the classroom, in the grocery store, on patient care rounds, or in committee hospital meetings. Some key concepts that can help us understand the dynamics of narratives are:

- **Narratives:** Often unexamined perspectives, cultural values, beliefs, and practices that are assumed to be the most common, "true," widely accepted, and influential within a given society.

- **Counternarratives:** Truths and experiences that arise from the vantage point of those who have been historically marginalized. These can either be a collection or individual experiences that run against the Dominant Narrative or dominant stereotype about their group.

- **Marginalized:** Excluded and ignored to the edges of mainstream society. Denied access to privileges and rights that dominant groups have access to.

Despite carrying many marginalized identities, we all subscribe to societal "norms," which in the United States set the tone for what is acceptable or expected of us. These norms become our "truths" and shape our conduct, defining what physique is "attractive" or "healthy," what mannerisms or dress are "professional," or what is considered a "family unit." The stories we learn and tell ourselves, either consciously or subconsciously, uphold existing societal power dynamics. It also influences who remains oppressed or socially marginalized in our environments, including healthcare. They are woven into our conversations and thoughts, and we often don't even realize we have them despite consciously feeling othered. Examples of dominant narratives that exist in the United States are *"mental health is a sign of weakness," "immigrants are lazy and are taking our jobs,"* or *"all you have to do is work hard and pull yourself up by your bootstraps if you want to succeed!"* I have often asked workshop attendees to reflect on what dominant narratives they have seen exist within their own organizations or educational communities. What values or norms are being prioritized or assumed in the workplace or classrooms? I recall one female physician educator emphatically stating, *"Oh, I know one! Once you become a mother, you compromise your chances of advancing to administration positions at the University."* This led a nursing faculty member to add, *"Or what about the angelic and subordinate nurse who is expected to sacrifice their own needs for the sake of the patient and are below other healthcare team members in the hierarchy of medicine?"*

When we reflect on the harmful beliefs and attitudes that these dominant messages uphold, we can start to see how they compromise achieving inclusive and equitable academic and healthcare environments. I would like you to reflect on one dominant narrative in your workplace or campus. Ask yourself, "How was this narrative passed along to me? How might I be passing it along to my trainees?" Now, consider which counter-narrative would challenge this dominant idea or belief, and think about how you can integrate this alternative perspective in your teaching or training program. If you're still struggling to grasp the concept of counternarratives, here are some examples of what they can sound like:

- Seeking help for mental health is a way to promote mental well-being, which is an integral part of overall health.
- It takes great strength to navigate new sociocultural landscapes and migrants can bring important cultural, innovative, and economic contributions to a society.

- The idea that becoming a mother hinders a career could be challenged by highlighting the leadership skills gained through motherhood, such as multitasking, compassion, and altruism.

A large area we will discuss in the third part of this book is how we can work toward decolonizing our curricula. This requires us first to recognize that Eurocentric or White-favoring/White-centered curricula in medical and allied health programs could uphold dominant narratives that manifest in various ways:

- **Curriculum emphasis:** Heavily focusing on diseases and medical practices that are more prevalent in Western societies, disregarding conditions and approaches that are prevalent in other parts of the world.
- **Historical context:** Overlooking or marginalizing the contributions of non-European cultures and civilizations to medical knowledge or treatment practices further reinforces the idea that medical progress is predominantly a Western achievement.
- **Representation:** Lacking diverse representation in teaching materials, textbooks, and examples used in lectures can reinforce the notion that medical expertise is primarily rooted in Eurocentric perspectives.
- **Clinical approach:** Allowing Eurocentric biases to influence the way various diseases are diagnosed and treated, potentially leading to misdiagnosis or ineffective treatments for patients from non-European backgrounds.
- **Language and communication:** When predominantly English-centric education is used, it can pose barriers for trainees who are English-language learners, potentially

disadvantaging them in understanding and performance in the program.

- **Research bias:** Conducting clinical research predominantly centered on White or male cohorts may lead to medical treatments and recommendations that are less effective or even harmful for people from different genders, races, or ethnicities.

Addressing these issues involves reforming medical education to embrace a more inclusive, diverse, and culturally sensitive approach that values all contributions to medical knowledge and prioritizes equitable patient care.

The Other Truths

Counternarratives invite a different "truth" to be told and heard, allowing us to understand the same facts of an event from the viewpoint of underrepresented groups. This becomes crucial in healthcare education if we want to enrich our educational content and conversations and promote equitable health outcomes for disadvantaged populations. Amplifying counternarratives can be through strategies such as:

- Promoting literacy and communication, fostering critical thinking and reflection in class, and inviting students who have been historically marginalized to share their thoughts first. Advocating for diverse voices and perspectives in media, literature, and other forms of communication is key to challenging one-sided narratives and fostering understanding across the field of medicine.

- Providing readings or literature about how social status, hierarchy, and a position of power influence the birth of dominant narratives in healthcare and education.

- Analyzing the source of biomedical information, identifying bias, and evaluating the credibility of medical or drug information would help enhance consciousness about dominant narratives.

- Considering the impact that dominant narratives have on a provider's thinking and action may inspire students to practice social responsibility and ethical principles when communicating with patients.

- Embedding storytelling and personal narratives as powerful tools for community organizing and social change. This approach highlights the importance of the stories we tell and how narratives shape our reality.

Examining Our Cycle of Socialization

I believe the Cycle of Socialization can help us and our learners gain greater self-awareness, have empathy for the diverse experiences of our patients, and promote honest discussions about social justice in healthcare. Developed by Professor Bobbie Harro, the cycle highlights how individuals are socialized into their roles as both oppressors and oppressed within societal structures. It emphasizes that breaking this cycle requires critical self-reflection, awareness of privilege and bias, and an active commitment to challenging and changing the norms and values that perpetuate inequalities. The process of internalized superiority involves people in the agent group adopting and displaying an unconscious or conscious belief in their own superiority, resulting in oppression toward both target and agent groups. In contrast, internalized oppression is when people in the target group adopt and exhibit feelings of inferiority, which can result in self-destructive coping mechanisms and oppression toward others in the target group. Internalized superiority and oppression are complex multigenerational socialization processes that can go

Chapter 5

unacknowledged and unaddressed if not recognized. As educators who are striving to cultivate equity and inclusion, I believe we should all examine the cycle and introspect. Consider the following questions:

- What are examples of socialization you have experienced in your personal and professional life?
- How might the cycle be linked to implicit or unconscious biases you hold about certain colleagues, students, or patients?
- What core emotions drive you to reinforce certain beliefs or values you hold?

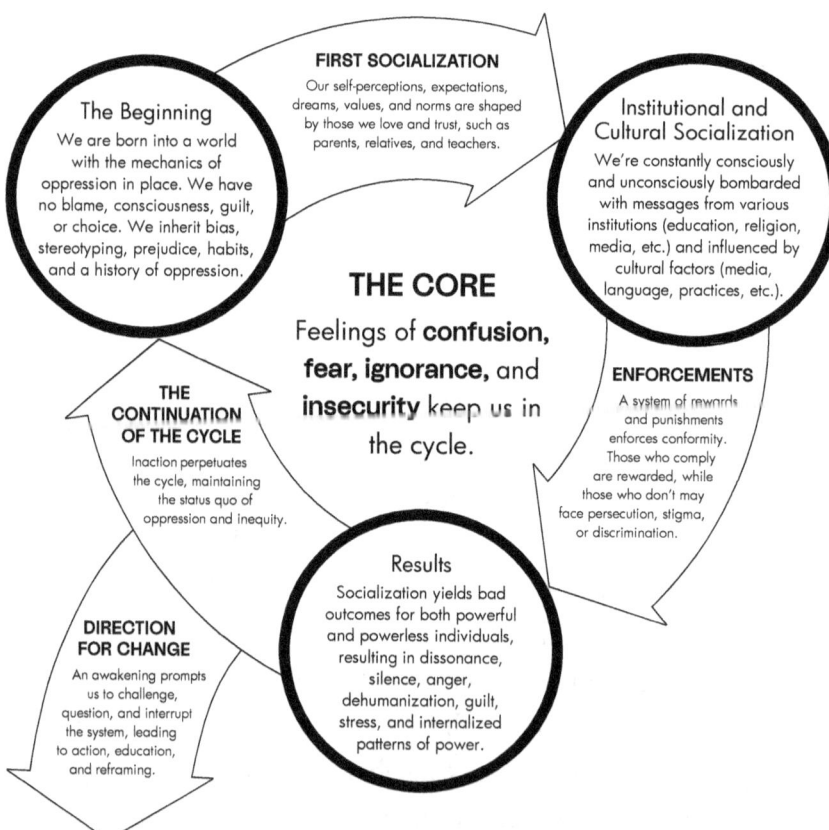

FIGURE 3: CYCLE OF SOCIALIZATION BY BOBBIE HARRO

Key Takeaways:

1. STEM fields often lack representation and inclusivity for underrepresented groups, leading to feelings of anxiety and exclusion among minority students.

2. Dominant narratives, shaped by societal norms, impact how we perceive ourselves and others, often reinforcing harmful beliefs and attitudes.

3. Counter-narratives provide alternative perspectives from historically marginalized groups, challenging dominant stereotypes.

4. Cycles of socialization help us to gain self-awareness and empathy toward others, while also recognizing and addressing internalized superiority and oppression in order to promote equity and inclusion.

PART II: THE PRINCIPLES

"If you want to change the world, first change your heart."
—Confucius

CHAPTER 6

•

The SHIFT Framework

*True inclusivity isn't about agreeing with everyone;
it's about respecting each other's differences
for the sake of our shared humanity.*

In ancient China, patients paid their doctors retainer fees if they stayed healthy. When an individual fell ill, these payments were halted until the doctor could restore their health. When I first learned about this model of healthcare, I was struck by how deeply it was rooted in a sense of humanity. It not only honored and centered health as the ultimate goal, but also the sacred relationship of respect between the patient and their clinician—the trust and partnership that was necessary for healing. In today's time, Western-healthcare systems should examine how we are misaligned to this focus if we want to shift our efforts to equity-conscious outcomes. So many of our health sciences carry oaths for a professional code of ethics that emphasizes humanity in patient care. While these oaths may not explicitly mention words like diversity, equity, and inclusion, they include the principles and values as fundamental to the provision of high-quality healthcare. Here are some examples of where principles of inclusion, justice, equity, and humanity may be implied in a sampling of oaths:

Chapter 6

Oath of a Pharmacist:

- "I will consider the welfare of humanity and relief of suffering my primary concerns."
- "I will embrace and advocate changes that improve patient care."
- "I will promote inclusion, embrace diversity, and advocate for justice to advance health equity."

The National Association of Social Workers (NASW) Code of Ethics:

- "The primary mission of the social work profession is to enhance human well-being and help meet the basic human needs of all people, with particular attention to the needs and empowerment of people who are vulnerable, oppressed, and living in poverty. Social workers are sensitive to cultural and ethnic diversity and strive to end discrimination, oppression, poverty, and other forms of social injustice."

Nightingale Pledge (for Nurses):

- "I will do all in my power to maintain and elevate the standard of my profession."
- "I will hold in confidence all personal matters committed to my keeping."

Dentist's Oath:

- "I will treat all my patients equally, without prejudice."
- "I will recognize my responsibility to society and will devote myself to the service of all humanity."

- "I shall respect the full human dignity of each individual regardless of their race, economic status or religion."

Hippocratic Oath (for Physicians):

- "I will remember that I remain a member of society with special obligations to all my fellow human beings."

Oath of Physician Assistants:

- "I will honor the diversity and individuality of all patients and will respect their beliefs, customs, and choices in the provision of care."
- "I will uphold the principles of equity, access, and fairness in healthcare, striving to eliminate disparities in health outcomes."

In addition to highlighting our duty to uphold such oaths, I also often tell my students we need to subscribe to the platinum rule, *"treat people the way they want to be treated,"* if we really want to address and eliminate the systematic disparities we see in healthcare education and patient care. This means that educators can't just instruct students to be inclusive; they must first engage in self-reflection and growth to genuinely embody inclusivity themselves. I believe that when we actively model inclusive behavior and create cultures where equity and respect are central to the learning experience, our students can see what this might look like in patient care. To achieve this, I propose the SHIFT framework as the core principles to reach our goals when putting into practice our equity-minded and inclusive approaches: **SHIFT: Self-reflect critically, Honor cultural and structural humility, Invite vulnerability and discomfort, Foster connection over content, Think active allyship and accountability.** Shifting our practices toward equity and inclusion means acknowledging the inherent dignity and human rights of every individual, regardless of their background, identity, or circumstances. It sets the tone that, as educators, we must shift our focus to creating environments where all patients and healthcare professionals feel valued, heard, and understood. I present these principles as anchors that we each hold in order to elevate inclusion and equity in our spaces:

Anchor 1 – Self-reflect critically: Healthcare education should encourage critical reflection and self-awareness among students, faculty, and staff. This involves examining our own biases and assumptions, as well as the broader social and political context in which healthcare is delivered.

Anchor 2 – Honor cultural and structural humility: Healthcare providers and educators must be aware of their own biases and assumptions, and continuously work to address them. By practicing cultural and structural humility, we better recognize and value the diversity of patients' experiences and the systems that uphold inequities that must be dismantled in order to promote equitable care.

Anchor 3 – Invite vulnerability and discomfort: Stepping outside our comfort zones, embracing discomfort, and practicing vulnerability can lead to deeper self-growth and foster empathy for the various challenges and experiences that diverse students face. This also creates an atmosphere of authenticity where students are shown how to share their thoughts, concerns, and ideas.

Anchor 4 – Foster connection over content: When we are prioritizing meaningful relationships, engagement, and interactions with our trainees (as well as among students themselves) over the sheer delivery of academic content, we essentially are emphasizing the importance of creating a supportive, inclusive, and collaborative learning environment that fosters deeper understanding, critical thinking, and personal growth.

Anchor 5 – Think active allyship and accountability: Allyship is a verb that must be put into daily practice. One way to do this is to ensure that access to healthcare education and services is equitable and independent of socioeconomic status or any other social determinants of health. Holding ourselves accountable for necessary actions is key.

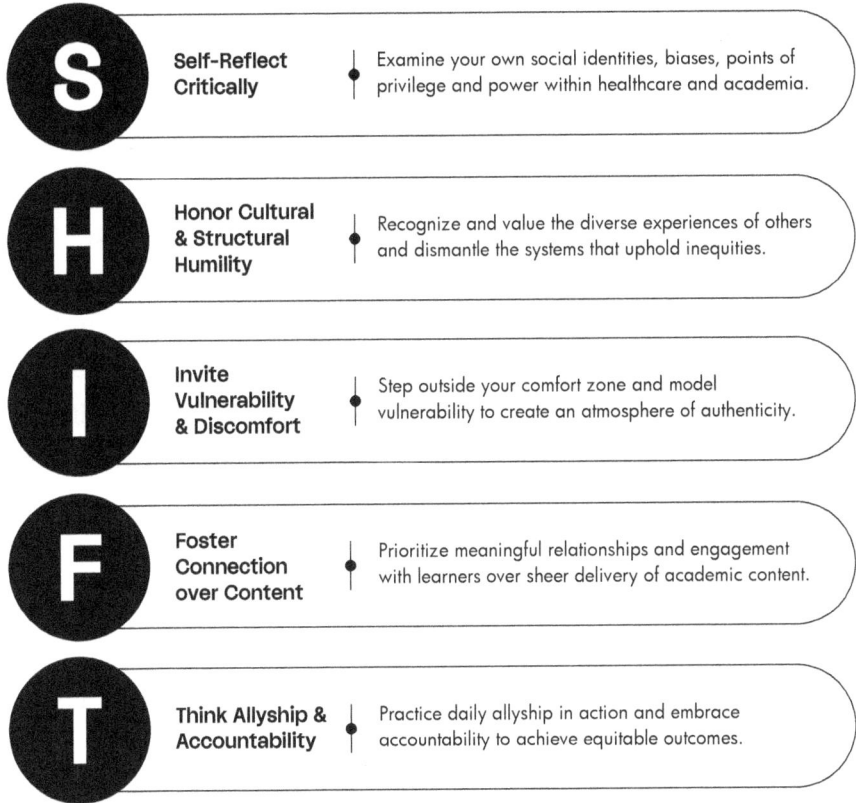

FIGURE 4: EQUITY-MINDED AND INCLUSIVE SHIFT FRAMEWORK

If we embrace these principles, our programs can be training grounds for our students and residents to thrive, not just survive.

Chapter 6

They can, in turn, create a more equitable and just healthcare system that meets the needs of all patients, regardless of their backgrounds or social status. Ultimately, implementing the **SHIFT** framework helps healthcare education programs create inclusive environments where all students feel valued and supported. This includes addressing discrimination and harassment, promoting diversity and inclusivity in curriculum and teaching, and providing appropriate accommodations for students with disabilities.

We have seen that the status quo in education often relies on traditional and outdated models that do not meet the needs of diverse learners, especially those from historically marginalized communities, such as low-income students, students of color, students with disabilities, undocumented students, queer students, and English language learners. To advance equity in education, each educator must challenge and transform the current system to achieve justice. This involves not only acknowledging systemic inequities—such as the unequal distribution of resources, inadequate instructor preparation, and bias in assessment and evaluation—but also taking action to address them.

Disrupting the status quo means challenging our own assumptions and beliefs about what education should be and who it should serve. I use the word "disrupt" intentionally because it signifies a shift away from "business as usual." This requires bravery. As discussed in Chapter 5, confronting the dominant narratives around us, challenging them, and amplifying often-overlooked perspectives and identities requires courage. Interrupting the status quo is essential for advancing equity in education and healthcare because our current systems are inherently unequal and perpetuate disparities in educational and health outcomes for students and patients.

All educators involved in shaping the future healthcare workforce play a role in reimagining and redesigning educational structures, policies, and practices to create a more inclusive, equitable, and just system. This requires actively listening to and valuing our students' perspectives, experiences, and knowledge.

In the remaining chapters of Part 2, I invite you to explore each component of the SHIFT framework. Reflect on what aspects you may already be implementing and consider how you can better prioritize and enhance these practices to create a more inclusive and equitable environment for your learners. By examining and refining your approach, you can make meaningful strides toward transforming your educational setting and advancing equity in healthcare education.

Key Takeaways:

1. Upholding our oaths for humanity in practice and subscribing to the platinum rule are essential for addressing systematic disparities in healthcare education and patient care.

2. The SHIFT framework (Self-reflection, Honor humility, Invite discomfort, Foster connection, and Think active allyship) serves as an anchor for promoting equity and inclusion in healthcare education—fostering environments where all feel valued, heard, and understood.

3. To advance equity in education, it is necessary for each educator to disrupt the status quo and actively listen to our learners in order to achieve justice.

CHAPTER 7

•

Self-Reflect Critically

"The unexamined life is not worth living."
—Socrates

While my professional identity centers around being a pharmacist and professor, I also identify as a straight, educated, able-bodied female. I come from a working-class immigrant Muslim family, and these aspects of my identity are crucial in influencing how I navigate the world and how the world perceives and interacts with me. This model is known in the world of sociology as a "social location." A social location is a combination of factors, including entities like pronouns, gender, race, social class, age, ability, religion, sexual orientation, education, and other forms of identity that shape how we see the world, access privilege or marginalization, determine our lens of bias, and even how we approach engaging in inclusion work. No two people share the same exact social locations—I like to call this our *diversity thumbprint*! We make fast friends with people who share similarities with us, but we make even deeper bonds when we know and appreciate our differences. We can hold multiple identities, and they can shift over time, which makes each of us unique in our identity makeup.

Chapter 7

Initially, as a new junior faculty member and clinician, I relied heavily on my professional title and rank when introducing myself to new students, residents, and colleagues. Like many others in healthcare, I was socialized to believe that these aspects of my identity were strongly tied to my sense of worth or value. Over time, I have transitioned to using a social location model with learners to demonstrate that the personal and social context of who we are is just as important as our professional roles or titles. Including my social location now allows me to self-identify and dispel any assumptions my audience might make about the visible parts of my identity. You know, the parts of our identity like race, gender, and physical attributes that walk in the door before the rest of us? It also allows me to center my humanity before my professional ranking. It sends a signal to my learners that, despite being a professor or a clinical pharmacist, I also carry many identities and lived circumstances that may not be visible. By doing this, it signals that I know my identities have impacted my experiences not only in my personal life, but also in my career as a healthcare professional and educator. It is critical for us not to disengage our identities with conversations around diversity, accessibility, equity, and inclusion. Now, take a moment to reflect on what your social locations are and write them down. How would you want to introduce yourself to others so as to dispel any assumptions about your lens into the world?

For many years, I didn't reflect on how the various facets of my identity influence my work as a healthcare professional, and ultimately, my ability to fully engage, be innovative, or advocate for my patients, students, and peers. Without exploring our social identities and how they lend themselves to power, privilege, and oppression, we can't move forward with meaningful action in the learning environments we create for our students or healthcare environments for our patients. There really isn't a way around this step, despite how often it is met with discomfort, confusion, or hesitation.

Examining Intersectionality

Intersectionality is a concept developed by legal scholar Kimberlé Crenshaw to explain how various forms of oppression (such as racism, sexism, homophobia, ableism, etc.) intersect and interact with each other, creating unique experiences of discrimination and marginalization for individuals who belong to multiple marginalized groups. According to Crenshaw, mainstream feminist and anti-discrimination approaches tend to focus on one form of oppression at a time rather than acknowledging the ways in which different forms of oppression intersect and compound each other. This approach can lead to the erasure of the experiences of individuals who face multiple and intersecting forms of discrimination. Intersectionality recognizes the complexity of identity and the interconnected nature of different forms of oppression. It highlights the importance of considering the experiences of individuals who belong to multiple marginalized groups and recognizes the need for a more inclusive and nuanced approach to social justice.

Change Starts with "I" and Exploring Your Identities

There is no single solution to address inequities, but a meaningful starting point is to explore our own identities. Understanding our own identities and their impact helps us recognize the challenges faced by others with different identities. At the same time, acknowledging our privileges enables us to empathize with those who have different experiences.

While identity work centers around "me," it is just as important for the "we" to belong to the collective spaces in which we deliver care or learn. In order to create inclusive spaces, we must always work on balancing identity, uniqueness, and collective belonging. If a learner or colleague does not feel a sense of their identities being respected and included within the collective, they are just another brick in the wall. Belonging is a sentiment that correlates with greater achievement, engagement, and effort. This is also where it is important to differentiate that "fitting in" is not the same as belonging. For example, if a student is told that they are part of a larger group, let's say a graduating medical class, but that their unique identities are not considered nor respected, then at best, we can only say we achieved assimilation. Expecting everyone to conform to the majority's norms is not the same as being truly inclusive.

Mapping Your Social Identities

"When we identify where our privilege intersects with somebody else's oppression, we'll find our opportunities to make real change." —Ijeoma Oluo

Social identity is a powerful force that drives the behaviors and roles that individuals are expected to perform. Culture also plays a role in how we socialize, practice patient care, and approach our own health. Culture can be described as the "sum of beliefs, practices, habits, likes, dislikes, norms, customs, rituals, and so forth that we learned from our families during years of socialization." Our cultural characteristics, attitudes, values, and beliefs guide how we experience health, healthcare, and our social identities. Often, healthcare professionals approach the medical care they provide to patients not only through their own cultural lens, but also their social identity. Our identity shapes how we see the world and how the world sees us. Social identities are used to categorize members into various groups such as race, ethnicity, age/generation, sexual orientation, nationality, (dis)ability, and socioeconomic status. While some aspects of our social identities are fluid or dynamic and change over time, some may stay static. Social identity differs from personal identity, which is made up of attributes you use to describe yourself, like being short or intuitive.

Social identity mapping is an important tool to uncover how our identities impact our teaching, care for patients, and ability to lead daily. It also allows us to determine where we hold historically marginalized identities (those who have had less access to resources and opportunities). Understanding ourselves helps us to know others better. Identities will help us to recognize when we are stereotyping. If we can catch our biases, it will prevent us from moving into prejudice or discrimination.

I invite you to take a moment to reflect on your own identities using the table on the next page as a guide. Keep in mind that this table is not meant to capture every category or example of dominant vs. marginalized identities. For instance, categories like marital status (married vs. widowed, single, divorced), religion (Christian vs. Muslim, Jewish, Hindu, Atheist, etc.), or ethnicity (European American vs. Latine, Persian, Hispanic, Arab, etc.) are not shown but still shape our lived experiences. This exercise encourages us to recognize how privilege and marginalization intersect in our lives, while appreciating the full complexity of identities extends beyond this table.

Chapter 7

Social Identity Mapping Activity

Instructions: For each social construct category select if you identify with dominant or marginalized membership.

SOCIAL CONSTRUCT	DOMINANT GROUP OR MEMBERS	HISTORICALLY MARGINALIZED GROUPS OR MEMBERS
Age	30s to 50s	Younger than 30; Older than 50
Race	White	African-American/Black; Asian; Hispanic; Native American; Pacific Islander, Biracial; Multiracial
Sex	Male	Female; Intersex
Gender Identity + Gender Expression	Identify with gender binary system: masculine or feminine	Gender non-conforming; Gender queer; Transgender
Sexual Orientation	Straight	Lesbian; Gay; Bisexual; Queer; Questioning
Socioeconomic Status (SES)	High or middle class/income	Lower income; Living in poverty
Education	Graduate or College degree; Private schooling	High school degree; GED; Public schooling
Languages	English as the Native Language	English is not the primary language, and may speak English with a foreign accent
Citizenship	Born as a citizen of the US	Born outside of the US; Immigrant; Undocumented
Ability	People without disabilities	People with physical, mental, emotional, or learning disabilities; People living with chronic illness
Body Size	Thin; Slender; Fits society's image of attractive, beautiful, handsome, athletic	Person of size; Perceived by others as too fat, tall, short; Unattractive, not athletic

Note: Table adapted from The Nova Collective™ Identity Mapping Activity.

After determining which identities fall into dominant or marginalized identities, ask yourself these questions:

- *Which identities are most important to you? Why?*
- *Which identities have the biggest impact on how others treat you? Why? Does your answer change depending on context (e.g., at work, with family, with your friends)?*
- *Which identities do you hide at work? Why?*
- *Which identities are you most proud of? Why?*
- *Which identities do you think the most about in your daily life? Why?*
- *What assumptions do you think other people make about you based on your social identities?*
- *What assumptions may you have made about other people based on their social identities?*

Once you start seeing how your social identities shape your access to resources, positions, or opportunities, you will start to notice how this impacts your students and patients. For example, which social identities are well represented in your classroom, professional organizations, patient population, or workforce at your healthcare institution? What is the makeup of social identities among the decision-makers in your faculty body or administration, and has this changed over time? When we better understand our own social identities, we can start to reflect on how to shift systems to have more consideration and empathy for those who are marginalized. We can shift ourselves into action when it comes to elevating equity-minded interventions in our institutions. If your institution is considering a new educational policy for students, what disadvantages could it present for students of color, students with disabilities, first-generation students, or non-binary students? Could it bring further burden onto students who carry social identities that would be more impacted, having downstream effects on academic performance or mental health? I encourage you to continue practicing critical self-reflection to promote equity and support the diverse needs of all learners.

Key Takeaways:

1. A social location is a combination of various identity factors that shape how we perceive the world, access privilege, and experience marginalization.

2. Intersectionality acknowledges how different forms of oppression intersect and compound each other and recognizes the need for a more inclusive approach to social justice.

3. Understanding one's own social identity helps in recognizing biases, prejudices, and stereotypes, leading to more empathetic and equitable interactions.

4. Considering the diverse social identities of students and patients is essential for creating inclusive learning and healthcare environments.

CHAPTER 8

•

Honor Cultural and Structural Humility

"Out beyond ideas of wrongdoing and right doing, there is a field. I'll meet you there."
—Rumi

Maria was a practicing cardiology nurse who found herself grappling with a humbling experience during an encounter with a transgender male patient. Chris was a newly established patient in her heart failure clinic. Maria's initial reaction upon greeting Chris was a mixture of uncertainty and worry. She had limited experience in working with transgender patients and realized that her lack of familiarity might hinder her ability to provide truly respectful care. Maria was, however, aware that patients who belong to sexual or gender minorities are more likely to be the recipients of discrimination in the healthcare system, to which she didn't want to contribute.

Prior to the appointment, Maria noticed that the electronic health record (EHR) had the patient's name listed as "Jessica," which added to her discomfort. Introducing herself, Maria felt a moment of hesitation, unsure of the appropriate way to address Chris. She stumbled over her words, catching herself before using the wrong pronouns. Feeling a pang of guilt for not being better prepared, she found herself tripping over terminology and second-guessing her explanations. However, she recognized that her discomfort stemmed from a lack of education and exposure, rather than any intent to disregard Chris's identity. Maria, determined to improve the situation, took a deep breath and addressed Chris before she left the room. *"Chris, I'm really sorry for the awkwardness earlier. I was thrown off by a different name in our medical records and realize that this might have been uncomfortable for you. I genuinely want to make your experience at our clinic as affirming as possible. Would you like to share if there are any specific ways we can make our interactions more supportive and comfortable for you?"* Chris responded with a smile, *"I'd be happy to. Thanks, I really appreciate you asking."* In this scenario, Maria expanded her lens and centered Chris' experience over her own discomfort. She realized that the practice of cultural humility could not be mastered in a single encounter.

If we are to draw a parallel between cultural humility and gardening, it's akin to a gardener appreciating and respecting the unique qualities of each plant. The gardener acknowledges the diverse needs of each species and tailors their approach based on the specific conditions of the soil, climate, and sunlight. In this analogy, individuals practicing cultural humility act as skilled gardeners—valuing the richness of diversity, fostering a deep understanding of various cultures, and consistently nurturing an environment where each cultural identity can thrive. Structural humility, in this context, is akin to the careful planning and organization of the garden's infrastructure. It involves creating pathways connecting different areas, ensuring equal access to sunlight and water sources, and supporting structures like trellises for climbing plants. The garden's structures are intentionally designed to accommodate the diverse needs of various plants, recognizing that each species requires different types of support to grow. Structural humility involves recognizing and addressing the systemic and institutional dimensions of inequities that affect marginalized groups to foster inclusivity and fairness. Cultural humility requires us to continuously learn, reflect, and actively listen when engaging with people from diverse backgrounds. It encourages individuals to approach others with genuine curiosity and a desire to understand their experiences and perspectives.

We know that empathy is an essential human quality and a core element of cultural humility. Empathy empowers healthcare professionals to establish meaningful connections with patients, providing crucial physical and emotional support to enhance whole-person care. Empathy also fosters trust between patients and healthcare providers, ultimately contributing to heightened patient satisfaction and the delivery of high-quality healthcare. However, it's disconcerting that words such as empathy, communication, and interpersonal relationship building (often deemed "soft skills") are sometimes overlooked by healthcare professionals and faculty. This oversight continues despite research showing a significant decline in empathy among medical students as they progress through their training—a trend not solely attributed to burnout. This should prompt us to question why these essential attributes are not central to what we model for our trainees, especially if we view them as crucial for building trusting relationships with our patients.

Let's talk about another barrier to the practice of cultural and structural humility. I call it the *"But, this is how we have always done it,"* argument. If only I could count all the times I have heard this as a response to needed change in our education and healthcare systems. The resistance to change and the determination to maintain the status quo, layered on top of reactive approaches to address difficult situations, make achieving equitable outcomes ever more

Chapter 8

challenging. Striving for excellence in teaching versus resisting (or even reacting defensively to) change are often at conflict with one another. For example, after teaching the same cardiology lectures for 15 years, I noticed a recent drop in student attendance at in-person lectures due to the availability of recorded sessions. A reactionary response driven by ego might be to think, *"I've always taught this way, and students used to come to class, so the problem must lie with them."* This could lead to implementing mandatory attendance measures to counteract the drop. However, a more thoughtful approach grounded in cultural humility would involve asking critical questions: *"What external factors might be affecting attendance that I haven't considered? Is there evidence linking attendance to performance? How can I incorporate student feedback to guide any changes I make?"* By addressing these questions, we can move beyond a defensive stance and develop more equity-driven solutions, fostering both personal growth and a more effective teaching practice.

Cultural humility involves embracing self-awareness, openness, and a willingness to understand and respect the cultural differences of others in interactions and relationships. It recognizes the limitations of one's own understanding and seeks to avoid making assumptions about others based on their cultural identities. It acknowledges we are not always the experts. In the pedagogy of the oppressed, Brazilian educator and philosopher Paulo Freire argues against the banking model of education as "an act of depositing, in which the students are the depositories, and the teacher is the depositor." Instead, Freire encourages educators to approach teaching with humility and partnership, challenging the traditional role of the teacher as the sole authority. He supports a collaborative educational model where both teachers and students jointly create knowledge and a more just world. As educators, we may not agree with or understand everything our students do, but at minimum, we must respect their dignity, humanity, and cultural identities, and backgrounds.

The concept of cultural humility also underpins developing an identity as a professional. A healthcare professional's identity must be internalized as they adopt the norms of their profession, thereby not just behaving like a doctor or nurse, for example, but also *feeling* like an integral part of their community of practice. Practicing cultural humility centers around critiquing such norms and developing how a professional thinks, feels, and acts when working alongside diverse social and personal identities.

Culturally Responsive Teaching

Cultural humility requires us to engage with others in a respectful and informed manner. But how can we put this into practice? Culturally responsive teaching and critical race theory can provide us with blueprints for understanding cultural differences and how systems of oppression, such as racism, intersect with education and healthcare.

In pharmacy education, it has been reported that most educators lack training when teaching culturally diverse students and, therefore, may struggle with understanding the cultural makeup of their student body. I could safely say this can be extrapolated to other health professions educators as well.

Culturally responsive teaching was first coined by Gloria Ladson-Billings in 1994 as an approach in K-12 education aimed at practicing cultural humility and promoting intercultural training for educators. Culturally responsive teaching is not a stand-alone course or lesson but rather a form of teaching that strives to create more equitable and inclusive classrooms. The following are five components that educators must employ, according to Winston and colleagues, when creating a culturally responsive learning environment:

1. Create opportunities for cultural socialization.
2. Adopt diverse teaching strategies to meet student needs.
3. Learn the cultural diversity of the classroom.
4. Develop culturally relevant curricula.
5. Demonstrate cultural compassion.

Gaining self-realization and proficiency in cultural competency models can enhance faculty confidence. Utilizing "Train-the-Trainer" opportunities could be a valuable strategy for programs to develop faculty and providers. Workshops and seminars on cultural competency have increased the perceived and documented ability to teach about cultural issues and diversity. Another strategy would be providing ongoing bias training to faculty and staff to gain awareness and enhance consciousness of issues that may impede assessment, admissions, and interactions with students or colleagues from diverse cultural backgrounds. The Intercultural Development Inventory (IDI) can be utilized to evaluate and assess cultural sensitivity and competence and can assist in curriculum planning and intervention design.

Embracing educator-driven and non-siloed experiences throughout the curriculum can, however, come with challenges and unfamiliarity. Improving the cultural competency of faculty and staff through training and education will not only prepare faculty to implement curricular integration of DEI concepts and practices, but it can also aid in the recruitment and retention of a more diverse student body and, as a result, increase the racial and ethnic diversity of the healthcare workforce. Enhancing student diversity can provide a rich environment for cross-cultural training and self-growth for faculty and students alike. Leveraging the cultural diversity of the students in the classroom can promote learning and connection between learner and teacher.

Critical Race Theory

> "The most difficult social problem in the matter of Negro health is the peculiar attitude of the nation toward the well-being of the race. There have ... been few other cases in the history of civilized peoples where human suffering has been viewed with such peculiar indifference."
> —W.E.B. Du Bois, Philadelphia Negro, 1899

What was W.E.B. Du Bois trying to teach us when he said this over a century ago? While it is upsetting that we are still working through racial disparities issues, I think he would be proud of our push to address racial inequities in healthcare—albeit we still have a long way to go to achieve true justice.

The often thorny and contentious topic of critical race theory (CRT), due to its misrepresentation in the media, was created to dismantle racial injustices. First described by law professor Kimberlé Crenshaw in 1991, its jurisprudential origins have now been applied to fields like healthcare and education. It entails educators to grapple with historical injustices while recognizing students' lived experiences, cultural knowledge, and worldviews. At the core of CRT is the question, *"How does racialization contribute to the problems we see in our healthcare system, higher education, or society at large?"* CRT, for example, helps us better understand how the gains of the civil rights movement were eroded in the 1980s and beyond. While CRT as a theoretical framework has been misconstrued in contemporary times, its relevance and application to teaching biomedical concepts are important if we want to implement clinical algorithms with a race-conscious approach.

When we teach about disease states, we often do so as if the body is a machine of malfunction divorced from external forces. Yes, we almost always mention risk factors and conditions that influence illnesses, e.g., smoking, obesity, or diabetes causing cardiovascular disease, but how often do we stress the impact of the imbalances of power structures, colonialism, and other systems of oppression that have infiltrated the way we practice medicine? CRT helps us teach our students about the upstream drivers that lead to negative social determinants of health, like lack of employment, housing, and transportation, that increase the likelihood of illness. Within our healthcare system, we see the intricate webs of health disparities, which patients often find themselves entangled in, unable to escape. Behind these webs are the "spiders," the entities that hold power to design and influence our healthcare systems, who thrive on factors like unequal wealth distribution, racial hierarchies, and disparities in labor and housing markets. Just as a web is not formed spontaneously, CRT highlights that racism and inequality are deeply ingrained in our society and fuel the building of the webs.

- **Racism serves the interests of the dominant group:** Racism benefits the group in power both materially and psychologically, maintaining their social and economic advantage.

- **Racism as a social construct:** Race is not an inherent biological reality but a socially constructed concept that shapes identities and power dynamics.

- **Differential racialization:** Based on historical contexts and social structures, different racial groups experience distinct forms of racism and oppression.

- **Intersectionality:** Individuals experience overlapping forms of oppression due to the intersections of their various social identities, such as race, gender, class, and more.

The Public Health Critical Race Praxis (PHCRP), which was developed by Chandra Ford and Collins Airhihenbuwa in 2010, was derived from critical race theory and gives us a race-conscious orientation to research interventions in four focused areas:

1. Contemporary patterns of racial relations
2. Knowledge production
3. Conceptualization and measurement
4. Action (e.g., implement solutions to reduce disparities)

Furthermore, there are eleven principles that link to one or more foci and can be integrated into interventions related to health disparities experienced by minoritized populations through a race-conscious lens: 1) race consciousness, 2) primacy of racialization, 3) race as a social construct, 4) gender as a social construct, 5) ordinariness of racism, 6) structural determinism, 7) social construction of knowledge, 8) critical approaches, 9) intersectionality, 10) disciplinary self-critique, and 11) voice. PHCRP and CRT also lend themselves to examining our social location (mentioned in the previous chapter), which refers to our position within a social hierarchy (e.g., privileged, marginalized, dominant, etc.) and informs how we perceive problems around us. For instance, when we are examining how to apply disciplinary actions to a student's case of academic misconduct, the general perspective is from the dominant viewpoint and can disproportionately affect a student from a marginalized group. CRT centers on the experiences of those not part of the mainstream and better allows decision-makers to understand their issues and eliminate any inequities.

As educators, we must recognize that much of our knowledge is outdated and upholds racist practices. At the same time, as educators who want to promote social justice and health equity, we recognize these are foundational principles of public health.

By implementing culturally responsive teaching strategies in both our curricula and pedagogy, we can promote intercultural development among our students, faculty, and preceptors. Investing in understanding critical race theory tenets and creating intentional training for faculty and preceptors on its application can enhance lifelong learning, promote racial equity in healthcare, and create best practices, even in resource-constrained situations. I encourage you to explore how both can support your ongoing journey in practicing cultural and structural humility.

Key Takeaways:

1. Empathy, communication, and building interpersonal relationships are vital for healthcare professionals in building trust with patients.

2. Cultural humility offers a practical and interpersonal approach for individuals to engage with others in a respectful and informed manner, promoting greater equity and social justice.

3. Culturally responsive teaching is an approach to creating more equitable and inclusive classrooms, while Critical Race Theory provides a broader structural and theoretical framework for understanding systemic racism.

CHAPTER 9

●

Invite Vulnerability and Discomfort

"The way to right wrongs is to turn the light of truth upon them."
—Ida B. Wells

I once responded to a student's question in class with, *"I don't know, great question. I will need to get back to you."* A more senior faculty member was in the room as a peer evaluator that day. To my surprise, I later found the following written on my peer-evaluation form: *"You should never admit you don't know something; you always know something more than your students. You don't want students to look down on you for not holding the necessary competency. As teachers, it's our job to know."* This feedback rattled me to my core. Beyond its blatant honesty, it didn't align with my value of humility. Isn't admitting that we don't know everything an important attribute to model for our learners? I've always believed this sends a signal that we, as educators, possess qualities like accountability, a growth mindset, and a willingness to persevere in the face of uncertainty. My response to the student in class that day was my effort to display my commitment to life-long learning. It was me putting aside my ego and the teacher-student hierarchy to fully lean into a shared learning partnership with my students.

Chapter 9

When did vulnerability in higher education become perceived as a weakness? I found myself reflecting on this question after hearing a medical faculty member ask me, *"How can I be vulnerable and still be credible in my students' or patients' eyes?"* after delivering a faculty development presentation. This question landed in such a poignant way as I realized that so many academics are socialized to feel that vulnerability compromises our ability to be competent in the eyes of our students. Where in our training did we learn this to be true? Credibility and vulnerability were never antonyms for one another, yet many educators have been conditioned to think so.

Vulnerability is a strength. But, somewhere along the way, higher education has standardized teaching and training practices to ensure consistency and predict student outcomes. This excessive focus on conformity has diminished our ability to practice vulnerability as part of our pedagogy. This, in turn, dehumanizes our learning environments and sends the implicit message that we must remove our personal stories from the curriculum. Although we know that mistakes and failures are essential for success, we often hesitate to share our own personal and professional challenges with our learners. I see vulnerability as holding elements of self-understanding, authenticity, empathy, and connection—qualities that we want to inculcate in our students as they strive to be the best healthcare professionals they can be. Vulnerability requires the systems at large to allow for the openness of mistakes that we can collectively learn from together and grace for experiences to be shared. Educators should feel that expressing vulnerability is an asset that enhances connection and builds trust with their students.

I once asked a group of students and residents to share the first word that came to mind when I mentioned "vulnerability." Their responses included words like "insecurity," "risk," "discomfort," and "being ridiculed." Displaying vulnerability is often associated with being weak. So many shy away from showing vulnerability due to fears of rejection and criticism for seeming weak. This discrepancy is quite interesting as research shows that vulnerability benefits our teaching environments. It humanizes the teacher to the student, leveling the playing ground. It is admirable and models bravery. It cultivates a sense of belonging and inclusivity. On the inside, it is considered weak, while on the outside, it is viewed as courageous. How can we embrace vulnerability as educators? How can we shift the perception of vulnerability to a positive connotation rather than a negative one without it being seen as a risk to our authority or credibility? I believe this requires framing vulnerability in the context of teaching and learning to be something that is modeled, celebrated, and honored.

Selective Vulnerability Builds Trust and Connection

Research indicates that when instructors struggle with vulnerability, it can impact their self-efficacy in the classroom. Embracing authenticity means we can be genuine teachers, fostering self-awareness and confidence without hiding our true selves. We transform by setting aside our armor and defenses to embrace vulnerability as a natural part of the inclusive teaching process. This does not mean we show or share all parts of ourselves, but perhaps practice *selective vulnerability* as culturally responsive teachers who share successes, failures, risks we've taken, and aspects of our personal identities that helped us achieve our goals as professionals. Over the years, when I asked my students, "*What makes you feel comfortable seeking assistance from a faculty member or trainer?*" I was often met with responses highlighting the lack of an authoritative tone, an openness to share who they are beyond their role as an educator or healthcare professional, or a shared sense of identity, whether it's across religion, race, or other factors of social identity. The use of selective vulnerability allows for trust to build and for the students to see themselves as partners in the learning process. A willingness to genuinely cultivate a positive learning environment for all of our students requires us to share our stories as a tool to teach and guide our students. When we do, we create spaces where learners feel safe to share ideas, express uncertainties, and bring their authentic selves to the learning process.

Learning Edges

Like many educators, I emphasize the importance of cultivating a growth mindset in my learners and extend this approach to my DEI trainings. This involves stepping out of our comfort zones and embracing discomfort to maximize learning. Psychologist Lev Vygotsky's "Learning Zone Model," widely adopted by DEI practitioners and educators, highlights the need for challenge in order to grow while cautioning against pushing ourselves into the panic zone, where learning stops. I encourage learners to aim for that sweet spot, or learning edge, where knowledge and skill mastery occur.

At the learning edge, I tell my students they will feel challenged but still capable—there's a balance of tension and curiosity that should fuel our motivation to push forward. To check if we've arrived at the learning zone, we can ask ourselves: *Am I struggling in a way that feels manageable? Can I see myself eventually mastering this skill or concept, despite some discomfort?*

Our goal is to create an environment where perspectives, experiences, and individuality can be freely shared, fostering a "brave space" that encourages open dialogue and self-challenge.

Invite Vulnerability and Discomfort

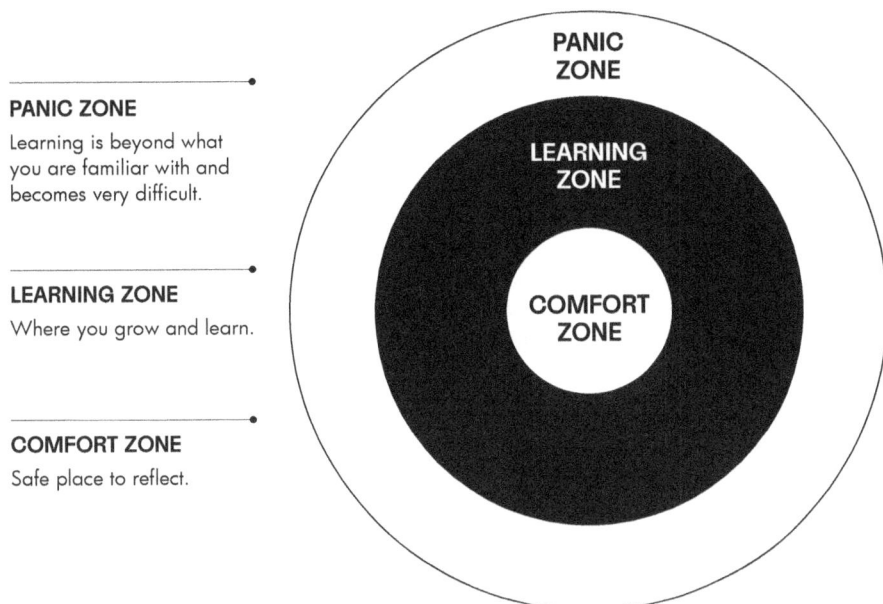

PANIC ZONE
Learning is beyond what you are familiar with and becomes very difficult.

LEARNING ZONE
Where you grow and learn.

COMFORT ZONE
Safe place to reflect.

FIGURE 5: LEARNING ZONE MODEL

We should strive to cultivate spaces of bravery, not just safety, allowing for collective exploration of diverse topics and genuine discourse on challenging subjects. In this process, we must also embrace that conflict and emotions like confusion, anxiety, frustration, and sadness may arise when we push ourselves to the learning edge.

I remember a moment in class when I mentioned Healthy People 2030 aims to reduce firearm-related deaths, acknowledging the devastating effects of gun violence as a public health issue. I shared with my students that, while I understood the statistics, I couldn't fully grasp the lived experience of growing up in a community where gun violence was a constant threat. When we, as educators, openly share our own learning edges with our students—now that's vulnerability.

Chapter 9

Center Yourself in Grace and Brace Yourself for Resistance

*"We may encounter many defeats
but we must not be defeated."*
—Maya Angelou

A conversation about vulnerability, mistakes, and discomfort is not complete without discussing how to extend grace to ourselves and others. Many individuals who find themselves leading or participating in DEI initiatives must see our call to action as a work in progress. We all start from a certain point and try to know and do better. We must allow ourselves room for missteps while acknowledging the importance of repair and correction. If we operate only from fear that we will do something wrong, we paralyze our progress. Building empathy comes from interacting with people who are not like us. Engaging with our students in ways that differ from what we are used to and are rooted in restorative justice is a necessary step to expanding our perspectives.

The work of transforming our systems is a team sport and cannot be done by just one individual. Any backlash should also be met as a team, even when the responses are targeting specific individuals. So, I invite you to reflect on your team approach—*how are you fostering collaboration and support in your inclusion or equity efforts?* I extend my gratitude to my global team of DEI practitioners and mentors, who have consistently supported me during moments of pushback.

As a gentle reminder to my fellow Black, Indigenous, and People of Color (BIPOC) educators and facilitators, we should recognize that we cannot discuss topics like inclusion, social justice, or equity without acknowledging resistance to change. I encourage us to name it. Name the tension. For the sake of liberation and equitable care, name the resistance that is fueling the reluctance to embrace change. We might encounter colleagues who, benefiting from their dominant privileges, view anything DEI-related as a threat and label them as "woke-liberalism" or "reverse racism." We may also encounter some individuals who only want to engage in performative allyship that makes them feel better or have strong desires to "save others" without undertaking the necessary self-reflection first. Witnessing these behaviors can be triggering and downright harmful. Yet, when we acknowledge our feelings, we pave the way for healing and gaining clarity. Conversations about systems and practices of oppression will always be challenging, bringing forth feelings of isolation, insecurity, anger, frustration, denial, grief, and analysis paralysis. We must hold space for all of it—all the feelings and all the perspectives—if we want to move toward a future of liberation rooted in compassion and healing.

Self-Care for the Change-maker

Advocating for equity, inclusion, and social justice in health professions programs can often feel isolating and challenging for many educators. Sometimes, progress will feel stalled. You may hit walls like I have when you feel a lack of willingness to take further action or push any harder. That little voice saying, *"What's the point?"* will creep in when we don't see any fruits of our labor or when hurdle after hurdle is thrown at us. Recently, a BIPOC colleague at a large medical center who is heading a DEI office said to me, *"I'm so tired of the White-washing, White-centering, and othering. I'm tired of stretching myself to fit in or being the source of comfort to everyone."* She had recently been tasked with securing a research grant for a project aimed at addressing the disproportionately high Black infant mortality rates in Philadelphia, to which she expressed, *"This work can feel so soul-sucking because sometimes I feel like I'm contributing*

Chapter 9

to the problem of infant mortality, instead of making it better. This is what happens when the boxes we operate within are themselves problematic." What her words screamed were, "*I'm tired, alone, and I've been asked to try to fix a broken system that is so much bigger than me.*" This work will test our stamina. It always has. Of course, we will get things wrong sometimes, or even get "punished" for taking risks. But just like the weather, some days will be sunny and full of progress, and others will be stormy and full of hurricanes that prohibit our movement and progress. When we center comfort as more important than everything else, we stifle our progress.

I often remind myself of the words of the American poet and activist Audre Lorde, "*Caring for myself is not self-indulgence, it is self-preservation and that is an act of political warfare.*" One of the biggest lessons I have learned is trusting and caring for myself, not just cognitively but somatically and spiritually. I believe that my well-being in this work is valid and a form of resistance. I am learning that if my body doesn't say "yes," then my mouth and mind should follow suit. The body holds the honesty we sometimes stamp out of our minds. Liberation is rooted in listening to our somatic messaging and reclaiming our thoughts of being in liberated relationships with one another. When there is trauma activation during DEI work, it is important to be aware of whether this is being dismissed, blamed, or minimized. We are socialized to prioritize our minds and intellect over our bodies. However, we need to shift away from this idea. I encourage you to explore somatic liberation strategies as a method for self-discovery and healing as you venture on your path. This might involve practices such as mindful movement (e.g., tai chi), grounding techniques (e.g., deep belly breathing), body scan meditation, self-compassion practices (e.g., positive affirmations), and creative expression (e.g., art and music) to alleviate stress and process emotions.

Key Takeaways:

1. Higher education has undermined vulnerability's place in teaching, hindering our ability to build authentic relationships, which is essential to nurture qualities like empathy, courage, and creativity in our future healthcare professionals.

2. When educators demonstrate vulnerability as a means to foster inclusive learning environments, progress might feel slow and uncomfortable, but is essential for meaningful change.

3. The Learning Zone Model encourages stepping out of our comfort zones and fostering 'brave spaces' for collective exploration of diverse topics and challenging subjects.

4. Vulnerability and discomfort require us to center grace for ourselves and extend compassion toward our progress and setbacks.

CHAPTER 10

•

Foster Connection over Content

"We need each other to know each other."
—Hakim Archuletta

We often say that a patient remembers *how* a provider made them feel during an encounter over *what* was said to them. I would argue that students feel the same about their instructors and preceptors. When we center connection over the content we teach, we can build compassionate relationships, amplify student perspectives, and make content relatable. Throughout my faculty career, the interpersonal awareness and confidence I had to gain to be able to identify how to have a constructive dialogue with students took immense practice. However, the payoff was rewarding—not only did I get to practice being a trauma-informed and culturally responsive educator, but I also learned how to co-construct the framework of classroom norms, fostering an environment for students' diverse experiences to be shared and validated. I'll dive into more details about these strategies in Part 3 of this book. These are essential elements of culturally affirming learning spaces, as they convince students that their well-being is just as important to us as their academic success. The bottom line is that we must prioritize connection over content. We have discussed how critical the feeling of belonging is to our learners. One of my teachers taught me that this feeling is exactly what compels people to join organizations, clubs, the National Rifle Association, or even cults. Humans have an intrinsic longing for shared experiences and connections with others.

So what are the elements of centering connection with learners and practicing inclusive pedagogy? It all starts with treating others' cultures and experiences with mutual respect and authentically validating students' lived experiences and identities. We must see diversity as an asset to learning, not a deficit, and integrate it into our classroom instruction. As educators, this involves not only understanding what students love, fear, and find exciting but also delving into their values, hopes, and dreams. Developing the ability to meet their needs requires gaining sensitivity to all dimensions of difference. Researcher Chris Hockings argued that *"inclusive learning and teaching in higher education refers to the ways in which pedagogy, curricula and assessment are designed to engage students in learning that is meaningful, relevant, and accessible to all."* Hockings also found that *"students value teaching that recognizes their individual academic and social identities and that addresses their particular learning needs and interests."* So, basically, our students are looking at us to create inclusive environments that reflect the people and the things that they value in our content in order for them to engage more deeply in learning. We also have to hold ourselves accountable, and our students must also hold us accountable. I continuously ask students to help me learn and help me reflect. I always hold space for exploring our social and personal identities in my courses and how the material intersects with our lived experiences. If there is a dissociation from the content, then distancing will occur, and belonging will diminish. I open the door for students to reflect on how their lived experiences are showing up as they interact with their peers, faculty, preceptors, and the campus community. A known barrier to inclusion and belonging in learning spaces is a lack of trusting connections with faculty and staff. Couple this with the pressure to meet high academic standards with limited psychological safety, and then we further compromise academic success. Additionally, *stereotype threat* exacerbates these challenges by causing individuals to internalize negative stereotypes about their social group, which can further undermine their performance, confidence, and overall academic experience. Research has shown that learners with marginalized identities—related to race, gender, or socioeconomic status—may underperform due to diminished self-concept, reduced participation in class, increased test anxiety, and lower retention rates if their experiences in higher education reinforce these negative stereotypes.

When we place a genuine emphasis on forging meaningful bonds, fostering active participation, and promoting positive interactions with trainees and students—we are essentially humanizing the training experience and creating a nurturing learning environment where our students can grow. Yes, gaining academic knowledge in subjects like anatomy, pathophysiology, and pharmacology is important, but this can be ignited when we center our connections with students to foster deeper understanding, critical thinking, and personal growth.

Students Are Not Objects of Learning

One of the most traditional perspectives on students is to see them as passive recipients of learning, wherein knowledge is deposited into their minds within a hierarchical system. In this model, we see communication can become one-sided, and it is not conscious of intentional connection and relationship building.

Chapter 10

Teachers pass along information, and students dutifully receive, memorize, and regurgitate it. Students are confined to the role of storage units, lacking true agency in the learning process. They are, in essence, denied an active role in their own education. What I propose is that we aim to see ourselves in partnership with our students and rather invest in creating a culture of compassion and conscious connection—where we intentionally create containers of psychological safety for them to bring their whole selves to the learning process. Victor Pereira, a Harvard Graduate School of Education Professor, said, *"Teaching with compassion means understanding their stories and taking the time to know yourself as we check our biases and lead with inquiry."* This means we prioritize asking students to share what their hopes, dreams, and barriers concerning their learning are. We intentionally create space to actively listen to their answers. *And we are willing to believe them.* Far too often, we take steps to open ourselves up to asking students, yet we fall short of listening with genuine interest in meeting them where they are.

When I first started deploying my pre-course questionnaire to better understand my learners' preferences, needs, and learning styles as they entered into their first didactic year, I was met with many students' comments like: *"I don't want to be judged by my professors or peers if I don't want to subspecialize or take on leadership roles," "I'm worried that I may miss opportunities to be engaged," "I want to be invited to share my ideas in class," "I appreciate faculty who provide flexibility with due dates,"* or *"Having a grace period on low-stake assignments really helps me not obsess about the grade and really gets me to focus on what I need to learn."* Rarely was there a student comment stating they wanted more material to learn or they felt that content delivery was the key to their success. In Part 3 of the book, I share how you can enable connection through structured course design, inclusive assessments, and other equity-minded activities. But in this chapter, I want to now focus on why so many of these strategies help our learners feel a sense of belonging and confidence. After I started really centering connection in my teaching, I started to receive student feedback stating they feel "comfortable," "enlightened," "aware," "more interested," "relaxed," "confident," "inspired," and "motivated" to engage with the material taught. Connecting with our learners, first and foremost, helps us better understand what matters to them through the lens of their existing identities and lived experiences. As educators who are also aware of their own social identities (see Chapter 7), we can also be cognizant that our identities can influence communication styles and preferences. Educators who are attuned to these differences can adapt their communication to better connect with students and ensure they feel heard and valued. On the flip side, when biases or stereotypes are not recognized based on social identities, this can truly hinder our ability to authentically connect with students. It is essential for educators to recognize and address these biases to build authentic connections.

Connection Feeds Systemic Changes for Equity

Several years into Course Directing, I encountered a student who was a veteran, a first-generation college student, and was struggling with weekly quizzes in my course. During my first visit with the student, I gathered it wasn't a competency deficit or study habit issue. During our second meeting, he gained the comfort of disclosing that he was living in his car with his spouse and 4-year-old daughter due to a bad financial investment when trying to put a down payment on a new home earlier that year. He was embarrassed, and I recognized the bravery it took for him to share his situation with me. I also knew this was not a situation that I could single-handedly help resolve. It required me to engage our financial aid, student services, and wellness office. Interpersonal connections with students are important, but the data we gather from our one-on-one conversations also beckons us to explore any disconnections within our institutions. In this case, I found out there were no clear structures in place for students struggling with housing or food-insecurity. I also learned that fostering inclusion is a collective responsibility.

To drive positive institutional change, many studies suggest using a combination of "top-down" and "bottom-up" strategies, departmental context awareness, and gathering robust evidence of the gaps. For instance, our students might share challenges such as navigating loan forgiveness programs, finding accessible mental health counseling, dealing with domestic violence, or addressing unmet disability accommodations. We have a responsibility to ask more questions to get central services and support systems involved. Think of using connection with students as a diversity barometer—a way to measure what's really going on. Or as a measure of our collective heartbeat based on resources being dedicated to creating an inclusive environment for learners. There is an importance to not engaging in the connection game in a silo as an educator. Our individual efforts to connect with our learners help inform a broader culture of inclusion. What we do as individuals is deeply connected to the bigger picture. A holistic institutional approach to create a culture change across the entire institution hinges on our individual desire to dig deeper into our connection with our students.

Stepping outside ourselves to gain new perspectives and learn about the diversity of our learners is an equity-minded approach that most students appreciate. It truly deepens the relationship-building needed in our health professions programs.

Key Takeaways:

1. When we prioritize connections over content, we are better able to focus on understanding students' stories through active listening, which fosters a sense of belonging.

2. Conventional models of seeing students as passive recipients of learning should shift toward a partnership where students' aspirations, barriers, and preferences are considered.

3. Our personal connections with students can unearth their struggles, which can instigate holistic institutional approaches that cultivate a culture of inclusion and positive transformation.

CHAPTER 11

•

Think Active Allyship

*"Our lives begin to end the day we become
silent about things that matter."*
—Martin Luther King Jr.

It was a Friday afternoon after a long week of teaching when I received an email from a medical student I had recently met during a visit to a Predominately White Institution (PWI), where I had been invited to speak about active allyship:

Hello Dr. Arif:

I am a second-year student on my school's social equity admissions committee. I was recently contacted to participate in a student video for my University. My face and likeness have been used before for Instagram etc. I can only assume it is in part due to being one of very few African Americans in the medical program.

I need your input on an email reply because if I am going to participate in such marketing, I'd like it not to be a false representation. Instead, I want to be a part of increasing diversity!

If you have any edits to my email reply below, ideas on how to leverage this opportunity or think I should turn it down, you can text or email me!

Chapter 11

> Reply Draft:
>
> Hello,
>
> I am interested in participating. I do not, however, want to give a false portrayal of the University's diversity. Instead, I hope that this video will be one step of many to help improve our school's racial and ethnic diversity.
>
> I would like to know if you have any information on how the University may plan to use this video or other info on diversity efforts.
>
> Best,
>
> Kiera

Kiera is a pseudonym used to safeguard the student's identity, but the email was all too real. In the post-2020 era, such communications have become increasingly common, prompting students to reflect on their role in diversity or inclusion efforts and the institution's authentic allyship. While I commend the student for prioritizing their values and addressing their needs in the situation, it also got me thinking about the responsibilities that individuals and institutions have to cultivating inclusion.

The role that authentic allyship plays in efforts to promote inclusion is important. I say "authentic" intentionally because allyship is a verb, not a noun. It is not a badge you wear. It is not a sticker on your office door. It is based on action and accountability. Allyship requires folks with dominant identities to recognize their privilege and be willing to share power to create inclusivity and equity in our educational and healthcare settings. This process is proactive and active, not passive. It requires one to challenge their prejudices and their discomforts to dedicate time, energy, and patience in the name of promoting change. This goes beyond just respecting one another or being kind to taking the responsibility and accountability to dismantle structures of inequities. An ally's actions are intentional and conscious. There is a willingness to transfer power to those who have historically been marginalized, a willingness to educate oneself and not wait to be educated. This process again starts with self-reflection by asking questions like: *What am I willing to disrupt in the current practices, policies, and systems around that present barriers in healthcare education? In patient care? What resources am I willing to dedicate to create meaningful changes to my daily actions to promote equity in my spheres of influence?* Hiding behind a shield of neutrality as a crutch to action should be faced head-on if we want to say we are allies. For example, if your institution claims to value cultural representation by encouraging students to see themselves reflected in the halls and walls, yet simultaneously enforces a graduation dress code that prohibits wearing culturally significant attire or items to honor their heritage during commencement, then this is merely performative lip service to celebrating diversity. Practicing allyship in this scenario involves advocating for inclusive policies that celebrate cultural identities.

Preventing Cultural Taxation

The term "Cultural Taxation" was coined by educator Amado Padilla in 1994 to describe the undue burden placed on minoritized academic faculty and staff, compelling them to educate others about their cultures, experiences, and perspectives, often without proper compensation or acknowledgment. Allyship becomes crucial in alleviating this cultural taxation, sometimes referred to as the "minority tax," associated with educating others on DEI initiatives. Allies play a vital role in ensuring that the responsibility for advocacy is not disproportionately placed on those already marginalized. For individuals holding minoritized identit(ies), attaining a leadership position often involves surpassing expectations and investing additional emotional labor. The prevalence of cultural taxation on minorities can exacerbate disparities in academic and healthcare

Chapter 11

leadership roles in the United States. For example, if a Black female academic is consistently asked to contribute to every resource group or committee focused on diversity and inclusion within her institution, it raises concerns about when she will find the opportunity to focus on her professional development or leadership skills beyond these roles.

Missteps Will Happen

I have seen people who carry many dominant identities, such as being White, able-bodied, cisgendered, heterosexual, and financially secure—who are recognized as holding most of the power in US society and globally—often worry about making mistakes when trying to be an ally. Many of these individuals, often in leadership positions within healthcare and educational institutions, express concerns about their approach when attempting to be true allies. Common sentiments include phrases like *"No one wants the white guy to talk about diversity"* or *"I'll just mess things up."* While mistakes may inevitably occur, the emphasis should be on repair and the various roles allies can fulfill. Plus missteps are opportunities to learn and lean into our practice of cultural humility. It's crucial to recognize that being an ally doesn't necessitate firsthand experience of historical oppression or marginalization. Instead, it requires a willingness to acknowledge the struggle and navigate any feelings of doubt, fear, shame, or guilt in order to take meaningful action.

Activist Leslie Mac has stated, *"The goal is not just to have people learn about white supremacy, but to understand how their personal lives support it. White people need to do a lot of introspective work to understand the ways in which they personally contribute to, benefit from, and tolerate white supremacy. This isn't about shame."*

Understanding and gaining the tools and strategies to learn how to be culturally sensitive enough to apologize and focus on the end goal of justice is important. Practicing empathy is a key component that drives a deeper understanding of others' struggles; getting to understand what motivates our learners, the aspirations of our colleagues, or the circumstances of one's experiences allows allies to build trust with the groups that they want to support. It's not about taking up space; it's about sharing space and passing the mic to those who often don't have the opportunity to speak. It is very easy to fall into a savior attitude when practicing allyship, and that is something that we should continuously audit for. While the intentions might be correct to step in and speak on behalf of someone being harassed or discriminated against, it must not be done as a rescue method or to appear progressive.

An ally that might hold power in hiring or promoting others should also consider being a sponsor for those from marginalized groups. A sponsor is someone who will say your name in a room that you are not in and advocate for you in institutional decision-making or career advancements. For example, a faculty member who is a sponsor to student leaders in the LGBTQ+ community who have generated ideas for cultivating safe spaces on campus would either invite these students to present their ideas to the faculty senate or share their ideas if the students don't feel comfortable attending. At such a meeting, this faculty member would amplify the voices of the students before they amplify their own voice of support. It is also important in this advocacy to take note of the nature of our allyship. Are we supporting the cause because we share an affinity with the group we are supporting? This is often called affinity bias. One should ask themselves: *Who have I been sponsoring in the past? What motivates me to sponsor these individuals? Do I share characteristics with them? Am I willing to sponsor individuals who have different upbringings, beliefs, and cultural backgrounds than myself?*

Chapter 11
Allyship Is a Daily Reset Button

I like to think of allyship as a daily reset button. A pause that gets us to think about the situations we are in day to day with a new lens of equity and inclusivity. Our goal is that everyone we work alongside, our students, colleagues, and patients, all feel respected and comfortable. As you push the reset button each day, ask yourself if you are striving to:

- Continuously reflect on the cost of staying silent.
- Take ownership of your own learning.
- Take ownership of your missteps or mistakes.
- Put aside your own agenda; no one is being asked to be "saved."
- Put aside your own intent in order to center others.

As healthcare professionals, we must root for practicing active allyship as part of our professional development. We must also recognize tha the contemporary settings of healthcare we practice within are rooted in unjust structures that produce health disparities.

The Coin Model of Privilege and Critical Allyship offers a framework for healthcare providers and patient advocates to navigate the privilege they hold. The coin serves as a representation of societal norms and patterns that bestow opportunities and privileges unequally. Each system of inequity, such as heterosexism, ableism, and racism, is likened to an individual coin. The top side of the coin symbolizes unearned privileges conferred based on certain identities or access to opportunities, while the bottom signifies the lack of opportunities, encompassing issues like inadequate healthcare access, discrimination, and under-resourced neighborhoods that many patients confront, resulting in health disparities.

As allies, our primary task is to become aware of our position on the top side of the coin and actively collaborate with those on the bottom to dismantle oppressive systems that create inequities. Depending on our social identities, we may need to assess our stance on both sides of the coin. For instance, as a female healthcare professional, I possess privileges when advocating for women's reproductive rights but may encounter disadvantages when pushing for policy reform or resource allocation within a patriarchal healthcare system. This model encourages reflection and engagement to promote equity and justice in healthcare.

Since allyship is not a badge but rather a verb rooted in action, we model our daily practice of allyship with our interactions with trainees and patients. Allyship is based on acting in solidarity with those who are on the bottom of the coin. Instead of thinking of patient problems as "their problems," we refocus this to "our problem" as we continuously work on viewing both sides of the coin. We must recognize our own roles in perpetuating systems of inequity in our healthcare environments and work in partnership with our patients and communities to create solutions to their healthcare needs. Critical allyship requires deep curiosity in getting to know more about others, not for the purpose of "saving them" but rather to work collectively to create social change.

Accountability Is Recognizing and Overcoming the Resistance to Take Action

"I want to do this right; I mean, I don't want to make unintentional mistakes or offend anyone. Sometimes it just feels like I'm walking through a landmine," expressed a faculty member who approached me after a seminar I conducted at a large university where I was invited to lead a faculty retreat. This sentiment was not unfamiliar to me, as I had heard similar concerns before. Educators

Chapter 11

and healthcare professionals are naturally inclined to prioritize the well-being of others. As high achievers, many of us can be hard on ourselves, constantly striving for excellence while juggling the demands of our roles. However, acknowledging that, as inherently flawed humans, we are bound to make mistakes despite our best intentions is crucial. It is important to approach allyship with an open mind, a willingness to learn, and a commitment to personal growth. Sometimes, there can be resistance to being an ally, which can stem from various psychological, societal, and personal factors. Recognizing these reasons for resistance can help us see barriers and then take steps to overcome them. When feeling resistance, pause and review this list to see why you may be hesitant to take action:

- **Fear of uncomfortable conversations:** Being an ally often involves engaging in difficult conversations about privilege, bias, and discrimination. These discussions can be uncomfortable and may challenge our existing beliefs and assumptions.

- **Personal identity and ego:** Acknowledging our privileges and biases can be threatening to our self-concept. It might lead to feelings of guilt, shame, or defensiveness, as we grapple with the idea that we might have unknowingly contributed to inequality.

- **Lack of awareness:** Sometimes, resistance arises due to a lack of awareness about the experiences and challenges faced by marginalized groups. Without understanding their perspective, it is difficult to recognize the need for allyship.

- **Social norms and peer pressure:** Societal norms and peer groups can play a role in resistance. We might fear backlash from those who hold different views or worry about standing out from the crowd.

- **Fear of making mistakes:** The fear of saying or doing something wrong can deter people from being allies. They might worry that their actions will be misinterpreted, causing harm rather than support.
- **Perceived threat:** Some individuals might adopt a zero-sum mindset, perceiving that supporting marginalized groups could threaten their own resources, opportunities, or social standing. This perception of competition can create resistance.
- **Comfort zone:** Stepping out of one's comfort zone and challenging one's beliefs requires effort and vulnerability. It is natural to resist change, especially when it involves self-examination.

Often, a paradox or contradiction seen in higher education lies in the way we strive to be thought leaders and catalysts for societal change while simultaneously tolerating shortcomings in social justice within our own academic institutions. I have found that finding a support system of "accountability allies" has helped me stay focused on my goals and serves as a sounding board for situations that arise. These individuals can be within your own institution or outside it. They provide an avenue for you to have frequent or scheduled check-ins to review situations and renew your commitment to your equity-minded goals.

Think Impact over Intent

A student named Carlos, who speaks English with a Spanish accent, was performing a patient exam in the dental training clinic. The supervising dentist, Dr. Thompson, was known for his dedication to creating a respectful clinical environment. After the patient encounter, Dr. Thompson, wanted to provide constructive feedback to Carlos about how to improve his explanation of a dental

Chapter 11

procedure to the patient. With the intent of providing guidance on effective patient communication, Dr. Thompson says, *"Make sure to speak clearly and confidently. Patients need to understand your points without any difficulties."*

Although Dr. Thompson intended to provide helpful advice on clear patient communication, Carlos perceived the impact of his words differently. Carlos, who already feels self-conscious about his Spanish accent, now worries that it might undermine his ability to communicate effectively with his future patients. He is left doubting his competency and questioning whether his accent is a barrier to his success. This unintentional microaggression, a subtle yet hurtful comment, undermines Carlos's confidence as a multilingual speaker.

This incident underscores a fundamental principle I encountered early in my DEI training—aligning intentions with impact. Regardless of our backgrounds or circumstances, it is crucial to create inclusive learning and work environments. The concept of *impact over intent* has become a cornerstone in my training sessions, workshops, and speaking engagements focused on implicit bias. It has also served as a guiding principle when fostering inclusive dialogue in my educational sessions with learners.

But what does impact over intent really mean? It boils down to—don't cause harm, and if you do, own up to it, rectify it, and don't center your intentions, especially when that harm lands on someone who had a historically marginalized identity or background. The idea emphasizes the importance of prioritizing the experiences and outcomes of marginalized individuals and communities rather than the intentions or beliefs of those in positions of privilege or power. It is based on recognizing that despite having good intentions, those in power may unknowingly perpetuate systemic inequalities and harm marginalized groups. As a result, focusing solely on intent can prevent progress toward equity and inclusion.

Carlos later approached Dr. Thompson in this scenario to discuss his feelings. He expressed how the comment made him feel insecure about his ability to communicate with future patients and that he felt his accent and language skills were being judged. Dr. Thompson was genuinely surprised by the impact of his words and apologized for not considering how his feedback might have been received. While the intent was to offer guidance on effective patient communication during a clinical encounter, the impact of the comment was the opposite, creating a microaggression that made Carlos feel self-conscious about his accent.

Putting Aside Our Egos and Defenses

Look, we are all going to make mistakes—it is inevitable. However, we must take these mistakes and turn them into learning moments. We can't let our pride or ego lead us in these moments. For example, when we step on someone's foot, we don't respond with "You shouldn't have had your foot there," or "Why are you being so sensitive? I didn't mean to hurt your feelings" but rather with "I'm sorry," and we try to be more careful. Hard stop. This doesn't mean that intent doesn't matter, especially when most educators and students mean to be compassionate and respectful of others. Still, it invites us to consider diverse perspectives and correct biased or oppressive comments.

The concept of *impact over intent* in DEI work originated from the fields of social justice and anti-oppression work, but it is particularly relevant in higher education, where students and faculty come from diverse backgrounds and have different needs, viewpoints, and experiences. Incorporating the principle of "impact over intent" can help ensure that higher education institutions are inclusive and supportive of all students, regardless of their background or identity. This means we must prioritize how our actions and words affect our

Chapter 11

trainees, rather than focusing solely on our intended goals. How might this concept look in our health professions programs?

- A faculty member intends to create a challenging learning environment to motivate students to work harder, but their approach may unintentionally disadvantage students who are not as academically prepared or do not have the same level of access to resources. To put impact over intent, the professor could consider alternative teaching methods or provide additional support to help all students succeed, especially those with neurodiversity.

- An educator intends to create a supportive course by telling students they are welcome to visit during set office hours after 5 PM. This could unintentionally alienate students who have family or work obligations after school hours. To put impact over intent, the educator could offer several times to meet with students both during and after school hours throughout the week. They could also offer meeting virtually.

- A professor intends to encourage critical thinking and debate over ethical medical cases in their class but does not provide ground rules for respectful engagement. The impact leads to unintentionally silencing marginalized voices or causing hostile interactions between students. To put impact over intent, the professor could model how to use guidelines or ground rules for respectful discussion, center diverse perspectives and counternarratives first, and proactively offer support for any interpersonal issues that may arise during group discussions.

In each of these examples, putting impact over intent involves recognizing that the outcomes of teaching practices matter more than the intentions behind them and taking action to ensure that all students feel included, supported, and able to succeed.

Key Takeaways:

1. Allyship is an active and intentional process that goes beyond just being respectful or kind and involves focusing on justice and empowering others rather than trying to "rescue" them.

2. Allyship requires continuous reflection, owning missteps, putting others first, and working toward equity and inclusivity in all interactions.

3. "Impact over intent" recognizes that despite good intentions, those in power may unknowingly perpetuate systemic inequalities and harm individuals historically marginalized.

PART III: THE PRACTICE

"A journey of a thousand miles must begin with a single step."
—*Lao Tzu*

CHAPTER 12

•

Moving Principles into Action

"Knowledge without action is wastefulness and action without knowledge is foolishness."

—Al-Ghazali

"I really believe DEI is important, but I just wish someone would tell me how to do it correctly," said a nurse during a training workshop I was facilitating. This was not the only time I heard a comment like this. This statement packs so many layers that need to be peeled back and examined. I am a self-proclaimed recovering perfectionist, and I know how to spot an "I got to get this right" mindset over a more progress-oriented mindset any day. The ever-daunting drive is not just about doing it "right" (as if there is only one way to cultivate inclusion and equity) but also about wanting to have mastery right away rather than realizing the need to find a starting point and pivot along the path to reach our goals of inclusion and equity. The statement also highlighted the far too often desire in healthcare and education to jump straight into the *"how to."* I get it. So many of us are juggling multiple demands as practitioners and educators. Let's roll up our sleeves and get to work, right? Many of us are "doers" and high achievers, and naturally, we want to jump straight into action. However, this mindset only contributes further

Chapter 12

to a checklist-oriented, performative approach to DEI work. We must resist check-boxing our way to solutions. Instead, we must learn to resist the instant gratification of "doing" and prioritize a thoughtful, mindful approach to achieving inclusive and equitable outcomes.

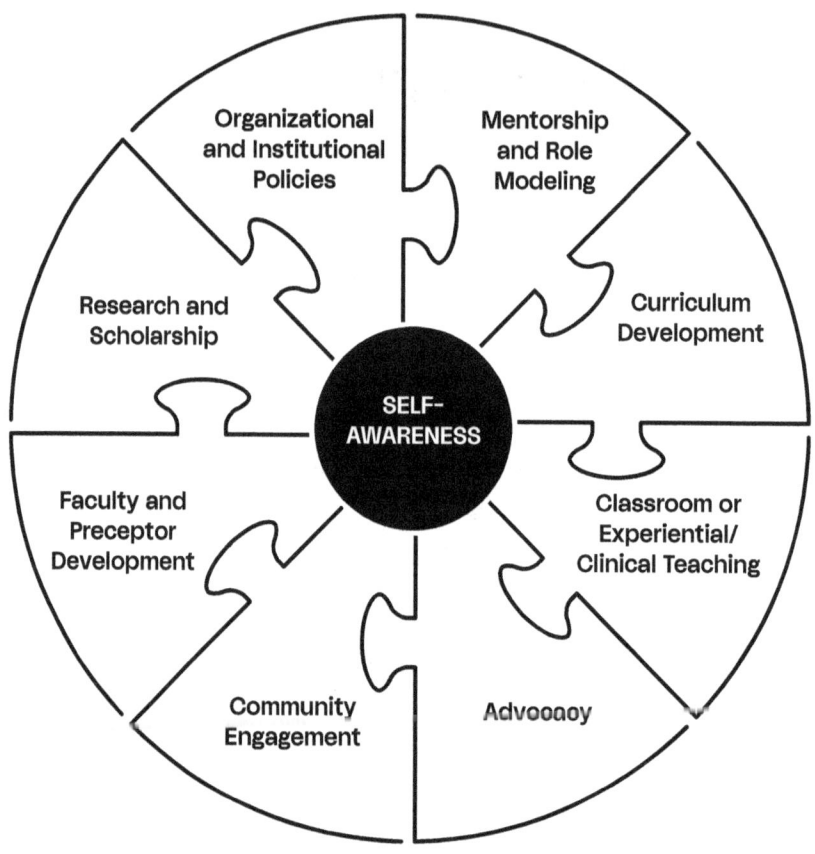

FIGURE 6: IDENTIFYING YOUR PIECE OF POWER TO INFLUENCE CHANGE

Successful DEI initiatives in healthcare and instruction must integrate principles into *intentional* and *strategic* action plans that are tied to goals. Procedural competencies are often very familiar

Moving Principles into Action

and comfortable to many of us in healthcare, but these only get us so far when aiming to embed inclusion into healthcare education programs. We must lean into our discomfort and aim to foster inclusive and equitable learning cultures where we don't operate from a one-size-fits-all-approach. Before jumping into putting the principles into action, consider how familiar you have gotten with the principles outlined in Part 2 of this book. Dedicating time to understanding the principles will provide you with a foundation from which to launch in Part 3.

If you are considering where to start, reflect on your role within your program or institution and identify your unique piece of power to drive change. Your impact will often depend on your specific role and the resources available to you. As you navigate the third part of this book, I want you to reflect on where you hold power and privilege to make real change happen. It can feel overwhelming trying to find where to start the shift to action, so ask yourself, "What spaces will allow me to best practice leadership in an inclusive and equity-minded manner?" Pick a piece of the puzzle and START! Don't feel you have to take it all on at once. Instead, here are some points to consider:

- **Self-awareness:** At the core of meaningful action lies self-awareness— an understanding of what we know and, equally important, what we do not know. Perhaps you're just beginning this journey, reading a book like this one to become more informed. Could you also share the knowledge you gain with your own colleagues and students to promote ongoing learning and improvement?
- **Curriculum development:** Do you have influence on curricular design or building educational materials to integrate diverse patient populations and cultural considerations?

- **Classroom or experiential/clinical teaching:** Are you an instructor ready to create an inclusive and equitable learning environment by promoting respectful dialogue, actively engaging with diverse perspectives, and addressing bias or discrimination in real time?

- **Mentorship and role modeling:** While many of us may be busy, we often officially or unofficially mentor students, residents, and fellows. If your mentees or trainees are from underrepresented backgrounds, ask yourself, *"Where can I further support their professional development by encouraging them to pursue leadership roles within healthcare?"* You can lead by example by modeling inclusive behavior, respecting diverse perspectives, and actively engaging in conversations about equity.

- **Faculty and preceptor development:** Advocate for training and development opportunities for educators. Leverage continuous hands-on workshops or discussions on cultural competence, bias awareness, and inclusive teaching practices.

- **Research and scholarship:** Conduct or support research on healthcare disparities, social determinants of health, and other DEI-related topics. Publish and present findings to contribute to the field's understanding and drive change.

- **Organizational and institutional policies:** Collaborate with administrators to influence and advocate for inclusive institutional policies. These policies can relate to recruitment, admissions, faculty diversity, and anti-discrimination measures.

- **Community engagement:** Foster partnerships with community organizations and underrepresented groups to promote health equity and improve healthcare access for under-resourced populations.

- **Advocacy:** Use your professional network, organizational membership, or even social media platforms to advocate for healthcare policies and practices that prioritize equity and inclusivity. Consider where you can participate in relevant committees or boards within your institution or professional associations to increase awareness and change.

Shifting to a more equity-minded and inclusive teaching practice includes a range of approaches considering the diverse needs, backgrounds, and lived experiences of all students. The shifts in our processes and procedures are to create learning environments where all students feel valued, sense belonging, and have equal access to learning. In order to do so, we must recognize and honor the cultural backgrounds, heritages, and differences of our learners.

While Part 3 provides approaches on how to implement change, it is not an exhaustive list. The goal is to offer practical insights that can inspire actionable steps—because every small action matters. It's okay if, as an individual educator, you still feel a bit uncertain about how to apply more macro-level systemic changes; these often require more complex decisions and involve multiple stakeholders.

In the first part of Part 3 (Chapters 13 to 22) of this book, we will explore how to put principles into action through instructor-led activities and instruction-based pedagogical approaches, such as:

- **Role modeling:** One of the most powerful ways to honor identity is through modeling empathy, compassion, and respect in our interactions with students, patients, and colleagues. We can inspire and encourage students to adopt similar attitudes and behaviors toward their patients by demonstrating these qualities.

- **Experiential learning:** Opportunities like simulation exercises, role-playing, and community service projects can provide students with spaces to develop their empathy and understanding for patients from diverse backgrounds. These experiences can help students learn to appreciate their patients' unique needs and circumstances and develop their individual strategies for compassionate and patient-centered approaches to care. Developing health equity content can help our students develop a more holistic and culturally sensitive approach to care that values the unique needs of each patient. When integrating health equity into our teaching, we must use a combination of strategies and approaches that help cultivate empathy, compassion, and respect in healthcare education and practice.

- **Reflective practices:** When we encourage students to reflect on their own biases and assumptions, as well as the broader social and political context in which healthcare is delivered, we create opportunities for self-awareness and growth. Encourage students to critically examine their own attitudes and behaviors toward patients to develop a deeper understanding of the importance of humanistic values in healthcare.

- **Intentional course design and pedagogy:** Using a "learner-centered" approach is important. This means having clear and measurable learning objectives and structures that take the guesswork out of learning for students. Providing access to knowledge and skill acquisition is a driver of equity-minded academic success. The use of modalities like equity-minded syllabi, assessments that combine low-stakes quizzes, various modes of teaching (e.g., gaming or videos), flexible due dates, and accessible technology are some strategies to implement instructional approaches that help our content reach all learners.

The second part of Part 3 (Chapters 23 through 26) will broaden our perspective of systemic and programmatic approaches to integrating equity-minded strategies into our curricula, culture, and climate. Ultimately, it takes both a grassroots and top-to-bottom approach to help ensure that future healthcare providers are equipped with the knowledge, skills, and attitudes necessary to deliver compassionate, person-centered care to all patients.

Key Takeaways:

1. When we prioritize thoughtful integration of inclusion and equity principles over instant action, we avoid being performative and foster more meaningful outcomes in healthcare education.

2. Regardless of where you move into action, be intentional about your plans, tie them to clear goals, and embrace any discomfort that may arise along the way.

3. Advancing equity in education involves leveraging our sphere of power to promote inclusive practices, such as through curriculum development, classroom teaching, mentorship, faculty development, research, policy advocacy, community engagement, and role modeling.

CHAPTER 13

•

Intentional Course Design

"Be a key that opens all the doors of goodness."
—Dr. Umar Faruq AbdAllah

No educator ever intends to leave any of their learners behind. After all, our success as teachers is defined by our learners' success, right? I can't count the times I have told my students and residents, *"I can't call myself a teacher if you're not learning."* This is why calling ourselves inclusive educators hinges so strongly on how willing we are to create and implement intentional structure and transparency into our learning environments and pedagogy. This approach encourages learners to bring their complete selves, encompassing diverse learning styles, into our classrooms, laboratories, and clinical learning environments. By transforming our learning spaces to be more equity-minded, we not only diversify enrollment but also create conditions for students to thrive. It demonstrates our commitment to genuinely accommodating each student in our courses—shifting away from a discouraging "weed out" tone to one that says, "You belong here, and I recognize your potential."

Structuring your course provides all students with a clear roadmap for learning. When the content is organized and well-defined, it eliminates guesswork for learners, ensuring that everyone can follow a logical progression toward academic success. This structured approach accommodates not just diverse learning styles but gives all students, regardless of their starting point, a clear direction on how to navigate the material effectively. Let's look at ways we can be intentional and transparent within our course structuring:

- **Class participation:** What might seem like an innocent occurrence of an instructor throwing out an open-ended question to a classroom of 100 medical students under the assumption that everyone feels equally safe and invited to answer is further from the truth. Most educators know exactly how this scene usually plays out. The same five students continue to be the first to raise their hands or call out a plausible answer to the instructor's questions. Structuring for equity could look like asking students to all answer using a polling question on the screen. Employ techniques such as "Think, Pair, Share" or encourage journaling prior to class discussions. These methods offer introverted learners the opportunity to contemplate their thoughts before engaging in conversation. This is another area to bring in "classroom norms," where students are asked to monitor their airtime when sharing. Or to encourage balanced participation during group discussions, you could ask students with two-syllable last names or those who speak more than three languages to share their ideas first. We can also strive to incorporate diverse perspectives and voices in course materials and readings to allow students from various backgrounds to see themselves reflected in the material or content.

- **Accessibility to course content:** Transparency in accessibility to our course content can also come through the modalities of technologies we use, whether that's Canvas, Blackboard, Zoom, or any other technology platforms. Equity means we assure that all students have proper access to these platforms, are familiar with them (*don't just assume they are because they are in a graduate program*), and have reliable internet connectivity to access digital resources effectively. A popular inclusive teaching framework, Universal Design for Learning, is based on providing flexible and accommodating support for diverse learning styles, abilities, and backgrounds. It involves providing multiple means of representation, engagement, and expression in the curriculum to ensure that all students can access and engage with the material.

- **Setting expectations on rotations:** Provide learners with guidance on what to do during moments of uncertainty (e.g., calling you on your cell phone if a patient needs urgent transfer) and for planned communication (e.g., meeting you at specific times or locations).

One of the fallacies I often hear from educators is that if we structure our teaching delivery and content, we might compromise the rigor of our courses or the students' ability to be "ready for the real world" because we are hand-holding them too much. This mindset also needs a shift. Research shows that when we fuel our pedagogy with a structured and inclusive design model, we actually help *all* of our learners, and those who might not need high levels of structure don't lose anything. The way we enhance structure and transparency in our teaching design is not just by clearly defining the learning objectives but also by blatantly highlighting these objectives when we address them within our content. For example, in my lecture handouts, I use a blue star symbol to highlight key learning objectives. The goal is to demystify where to focus and to minimize the energy our students spend deciphering the layout of our content. We want that energy spent on learning rather than getting caught up in how each professor organizes their instructional materials and resources.

Consistency is key when standardizing our format across courses in a curriculum, whether the course is biochemistry or pharmacology. This strategy provides a more user-friendly learning experience that aims to reduce confusion, streamline the learning process, and allow students to focus on mastering the content rather than grappling with different formats. Here are some strategies you can implement:

- **Use a consistent lecture layout and uniform naming conventions:** Maintain a standardized layout for handouts in a series of lectures, including learning objectives, epidemiology, therapeutics, etc. Use a consistent naming convention for module titles, headings, and subheadings. This makes it easier for students to locate specific topics and understand the hierarchy of information and what to expect in each section.

- **Adopt consistency in your online course platform:** Adopt a consistent color scheme and design elements within the course page. This visual consistency creates a cohesive look and reinforces a sense of continuity for students moving from one module to the next. Using consistent navigation tools, such as menus, buttons, or links, across all modules also allows students to easily move between sections with minimal confusion. Providing a clearly outlined timeline or schedule for each module in a standardized format helps students manage their time effectively and know what to expect in terms of workload and deadlines.

- **Standardize your assessments:** Be transparent with question types and instructions. This could also be done by outlining transparent grading criteria and rubrics for assignments and assessments to help learners understand how they will be evaluated and what is expected of them (more to come in Chapter 15). This helps students to focus on demonstrating their knowledge rather than deciphering new assessment structures.

- **Provide clear feedback and communication:** Establish a standardized system for providing feedback and communication channels between you and the students. This clarity helps students understand where to find feedback, how to seek help, and what to expect in terms of instructor communication.

Employing Narrative Medicine

During a conference keynote where I polled a healthcare educator audience, I asked, "Raise your hand if you enjoy using reflection activities as a teaching tool." In a room of nearly 400 attendees from across the country, only four individuals raised their hands. This lack of enthusiasm didn't surprise me. In the sciences, there's often a limited appreciation for and understanding of the effective use of self-reflection as a learning tool. It took several years into my teaching journey before I discovered the value of narrative medicine as a strategy to broaden my students' perspectives and self-awareness, emphasizing that illness and healthcare encompass not only biological or technical aspects, but also personal and social dimensions. I haven't looked back since. By incorporating narratives into healthcare practice and teaching, we can aim to improve

Chapter 13

patient-centered care, enhance healthcare communication, and foster empathy and understanding between healthcare providers and patients.

Narrative medicine is an interdisciplinary approach that combines the principles of literary theory, humanities, and medicine. It emphasizes the importance of understanding the social and cultural contexts of patient care to foster connection, compassion, and empathy. In narrative medicine, healthcare professionals are encouraged to listen to and interpret patients' stories to gain a deeper appreciation of their experiences, perspectives, and emotions.

We all have a story to tell. Narrative medicine emphasizes the power of storytelling for both patients and healthcare professionals. It acknowledges that narratives can shape how individuals perceive and make meaning of their health-related experiences. Behind every statistic is a human story. By sharing patient experiences, we humanize the data and bring a personal dimension to healthcare challenges faced by our patients. It's one thing to say social determinants of health exist, it's another to allow patients to share how these social drivers impact their day-to-day lives. Hearing first-hand stories about patients and communities helps break down stereotypes and biases. It encourages our learners to see patients as individuals with unique experiences. Through narrative techniques, such as reflective writing, close reading of texts, and group discussions, learners can explore and reflect upon their own experiences and biases, fostering self-awareness and empathy.

During a discussion in my public health course about the role of epigenetics, negative social determinants of health, and disadvantaged neighborhoods, students were allowed to share their stories. One of the few Black female students in class, Chay, shared hers with the class one year. She explained that her mother grew up

Intentional Course Design

taking two buses to get to school, and she only had to take one. Her father's options as a young adult were either to join a gang or work as a mechanic. She wanted her peers to get a glimpse into the decisions that were part of her family's journey to get her to a position where she could apply to graduate school. When Chay finished sharing, she was met with applause from the class. Later, I asked her how she felt, and she took a deep breath and then said, "Like a weight was lifted. I was finally seen."

By integrating reflective exercises like narrative medicine into medical education and clinical practice, healthcare professionals can develop a more holistic approach to patient care. It encourages a deeper understanding of the social, cultural, and emotional contexts in which illness and healing occur, ultimately promoting more effective and compassionate healthcare delivery.

Case Study: Approaching a Reflective Narrative Assignment with Intention and Structure

During my Cultural Care and Public Health course, I expect my students to write several short narrative reflections to express their unique perspectives, experiences, and insights. This personal expression contributes to a diverse tapestry of voices within my learning environment and fosters a sense of inclusion. While we know that reflective writing is a valuable tool and an excellent opportunity for students to think about connections between their learning, their past experiences, and their future actions, the question is—how do we structure it to be intentional and transparent? The first step is to dedicate the time and space to explain the purpose of the activity. Prior to the first assignment, I convey both verbally and in writing that reflective writing requires one to "re-live" an experience by reviewing the "facts" of what happened as well as their actions and feelings at the moment and then contemplate the impact of the experience on their future as a healthcare professional. By reflecting

Chapter 13

and then writing about these moments, it is hoped that each learning experience becomes more meaningful and will positively impact the student's future learning.

I relay to my students that there is no single way to prepare a reflection piece, fostering the idea of flexibility. The *"What? So what? Now what?"* model proposed by Professor Gary Rolfe and colleagues in their book *Framework for Reflective Practice* is one you can share with students as a framework for reflective narratives. Other authors have termed the three parts as background, relevance, and impact. The first part needs to indicate the evidence, the middle needs to discuss the principle on which the experience is based, and the third part needs to take a glimpse into the impact on their future.

Following a lecture and in-class patient case discussion, here's how I structured my instructions to students for a reflective narrative assignment using the prompt, *"How does race-based medicine contribute to misdiagnosis and mistreatment of patients who are racially minoritized?"*

What?

The first part of your narrative is factual information. The data, if you will. Imagine you're a journalist reporting the news, and you need to include in your data-gathering process: what happened, who was involved, when it happened, what surprised you, what was most difficult to grasp, and what others were doing at the time. You could say that this is the "who, what, when, where, and why" of your writing. You should include sufficient information so that the reader can feel as if they were observing the scene alongside you at the moment. It is imperative that you include evidence of the activity/lecture/learning points. For this prompt, you could describe how you experienced learning about race-based medicine in class today.

So what?
This section should place the "what" into a broader thought or a concept as to what you are learning in the course overall, other courses you've taken, or your past/future experiences. Think about why writing about this activity is important. You could state that this section describes the "relevance" of the activity. You should clearly indicate what you expected or anticipated about the experience and what you actually experienced or "felt" about the experience. In this section, you should be discussing "I" statements, such as "I believed this" or "I felt that." In other words, this must be personal, not theoretical or global. For this prompt, you could describe how operating from a race-based medicine viewpoint had impacted your community or gaps in your own knowledge.

Now what?
The final section (or "impact/plan of action") describes what you will do next based on what you learned from this experience. You might write about a new plan for the future, or you might state that "I now believe such and such" or "If I could turn the clock back to the beginning of the activity, I would do X rather than Y." You also need to connect the activity to the future—meaning, describe the way in which you will take this experience to your next stage of being a student pharmacist or the ultimate stage of being a pharmacist. Once again, you should be writing "I" statements, as this is personal to you! For this prompt, this could be focused on how switching from a "race-based" to more of a "race-conscious" approach to clinical care could contribute to more equitable patient care outcomes.

I provide the students with the grading rubric upfront, which outlines how a highly subjective piece of writing will be objectively graded. I also clarify how grace will be extended for deadlines on each narrative assignment through a clearly defined statement on the student online submission portal, as stated here: *"Life happens. A grace period of 12 hours will be given for reflective assignments that are due at 11:59 pm the day of class. The grace period is from 12:00 am – 12:00 pm immediately following the due date/time for the narrative assignment. If the grace period is missed, the score will be a zero for this assignment."* If I have multiple grading instructors in my course, we will proactively meet to discuss how to maximize our integrated reliability and how points will be awarded for each component of the rubric. And lastly, reflective assignments should not be assigned without building in formative feedback for the learner. There is nothing more frustrating and off-putting than to pour their thoughts and feelings onto a page for a grade and never receive insights about how their reflections were perceived by the instructor.

Key Takeaways:

1. Inclusive teaching is essential for creating an inviting and equitable learning environment. Instructors should be intentional in structuring their classrooms to accommodate various learning styles and ensure that all students feel safe and encouraged to participate.

2. Narrative medicine is an interdisciplinary approach that combines the principles of literary theory, humanities, and medicine.

3. Reflective activities encourage learners to make connections between what they have learned, their past experiences, and future actions.

CHAPTER 14

•

Equity-Minded Syllabus Development

> *"He who is illumined in the beginning*
> *is illumined in the end."*
> —Ibn Ata'illah

When I first started my teaching career, I was told that a syllabus is a contract between the student and their course instructor. I came to see it is so much more than that. It is a powerful tool that can communicate your equity-minded approach to inclusive teaching. When we review our syllabi, we must critically and systematically reflect on our teaching principles and learn to make inquiry a key and routine aspect of our educational practice. By creating a more equity-minded syllabus, we are not, by default, stripping away policies and rules. Having policies and rules plays an important role in supporting the structure of our institutions and our classrooms. Yet, when we only focus on the "rules of being a student," we are not able to look holistically at the values and tone of our course that are communicated through our syllabus. Our goal should be that our course policies and rules don't overshadow other content that is important to our students' academic success, such as resources and support services.

In order to maximize student engagement with your syllabus, go through the exercise of asking, *Does my syllabus:*

- *allow students to continually interact with the document because it is well-organized and easy to navigate?*
- *include language and tone that is respectful, inviting, and address the student as a competent and engaged learner?*
- *foster positive intrinsic motivation, one that promotes a learning orientation instead of performance (i.e., avoids focusing mostly on consequences, punishments, and scores)?*
- *include evidence that the instructor will support and incorporate all learners' backgrounds, identities, and viewpoints including when those differ from the instructor?*
- *include indicators that inclusive pedagogical approaches will be used?*
- *encourage the learner to connect with the instructor about course content?*

First impressions are everything, they say. According to pedagogical research, this applies to how approachable an instructor comes across through their syllabus. Furthermore, research focused on the experiences of students of color in higher education found that having faculty support is an important determinant of overall satisfaction and academic success as compared to White students. This means we must audit the tone and beliefs that are being communicated to students through the language in which our policies and rules are written. If I were a student reading my own syllabus, what impression would I have of the support provided by the instructor? Of the class environment they are building? Or even of the healthcare program in general? When we strive to have a more "learner-centered voice" in our syllabus, we can better focus on students' experiences throughout the course rather than just on the instructor's role. In this, we can evaluate if we are using "cold" tones, which are more punitive, versus "warm" tones that support the students in their experience. For example, a cold tone would sound like: *"Exams make-ups are not allowed without documentation of illness or death."* Meanwhile, a warm tone would state something like: *"Life happens. Traumatic events like death or illness are expected but unfortunate. Please get in touch with me within 24 hours with documentation so we can arrange for a make-up exam."*

Other areas to screen for equity-mindedness in your syllabus can include the use of gendered language or images. Masculine-wording and feminine-wording or gendered pronouns can be replaced with words like "you" and "they" instead. Commanding voice can also be evaluated by counting how often "student will" language is used and replacing this with more choice-based language like "student may" or "student can" to allow students to see they have agency and respect as partners in learning.

Accessibility to you as a course director, instructor, or preceptor is crucial to ensure inclusion—not only within the syllabus but also in your email signature. You can include easy-to-find hyperlinks to schedule meetings during office hours or list alternative ways to contact you (via phone or other virtual communication platforms) in your signature line. This simplifies communication and eliminates the need for back-and-forth messages to find the best time to meet. You can also rebrand your "office hours" to "student hours" to eliminate any stigma or negative perceptions of traditional office hours being only used for struggling students. One accessibility-enhancing activity is to invite new students to schedule a one-on-one meeting at the start of the course, where they can share recommendations for a book, podcast, show, or movie with you. This approach helps build rapport, demonstrates that you value their diverse interests and viewpoints, and, as a bonus, helps them learn where your office is located!

When you include a clear inclusion statement at the beginning of your syllabus this shows your commitment to respecting all students and viewing diversity as an asset, not deficit, in your course. Here is an example of a statement I use in my syllabi:

"My intent is for all students from diverse backgrounds to be well served by this course. My goal is for this course to be a safe and brave space for all students where all learning needs will be honored. I view the diversity that students bring to this course as a resource, strength, and benefit. It is my intent to present materials and activities that are respectful of diversity, not limited to gender, sexuality, disability, age, socioeconomic status, ethnicity, race, and cultural backgrounds. Your suggestions are always encouraged and appreciated. Please let me know ways to improve the effectiveness of the course, for you personally or for other students. If you may need any religious or disability accommodations that have not been previously coordinated, please let me know so that we can make arrangements for you."

Frameworks and Tools for Equity-Minded Syllabi

When we reevaluate our syllabi, we can practice social justice in real time. The *Social Justice Syllabus Design Tool* (SJSDT)—developed through a review of syllabi best practices, stereotype threat interventions, and social justice pedagogy principles—is an integrative framework emphasizing teaching that addresses power dynamics, reduces stereotype threat, employs diverse pedagogical strategies to foster belonging, models inclusivity, and connects course content to students' lives. This approach acknowledges students' diverse experiences and expectations, recognizing any potential anxieties triggered by the content. It asserts an ethical responsibility for instructors to create a classroom experience that prioritizes student success through both content and pedagogical strategies.

The *Center for Urban Education* (CUE) leads socially conscious research and develops tools for institutions of higher education to produce equity in outcomes. I recommend looking through their resources for strategies as you review your syllabus. When we embrace a growth mindset and practice cultural humility while crafting our syllabus, we allow ourselves to prioritize the learning process and acknowledge how our efforts can contribute to student development. It is essential to recognize that an instructor's mindset significantly influences the mindsets adopted by the students and their ability to overcome academic challenges.

Key Takeaways:

1. Syllabi should be seen as more than contracts, as they can be powerful tools for conveying equity-minded teaching.

2. Adopting a "learner-centered voice" in syllabi, with warm and supportive language, positively impacts students' perceptions of instructor support, the class environment, and the healthcare program.

3. Ensuring equity-mindedness involves screening your syllabus for gender-neutral language, choice-based language, and easy accessibility.

4. Integrating a inclusion statement upfront reinforces a commitment to inclusivity in syllabus design.

CHAPTER 15

●

Equity-Minded Assessments

*"When a flower doesn't bloom, you fix the
environment in which it grows, not the flower."*
—Alexander Den Heijer

I heard a tap at my open door at the college one morning. "Hey, we have to talk. All the students are cheating in our workshops," said one of the instructors in my team-taught course. "*I just came back from facilitating a workshop session, and most of the students are gaming the system by taking their laptops outside of the classroom to take the summative quiz. We must take action and let them know we're onto them. I think we should make them all stay in their seats until the end of the next workshop, even if they are done early with the quiz.*" I sensed the frustration and urgency in their voice. I was also not surprised. This type of response is common and reflects a lack of familiarity with the concepts of equity-minded education—an approach I, too, once took before I gained a deeper understanding of these principles. We educators often have a knee-jerk reaction to academic misconduct and want to quickly change our procedures and exert a zero-tolerance stance. This scenario has played itself out countless times across so many college campuses. Each time is like playing whack-a-mole to extinguish the academic dishonesty for it only to pop up in another way.

I now understand that equity-minded assessments are meant to uphold fairness and integrity. So many questions swirled through my mind as I listened to my colleague relay their concerns and potential solutions. Are we modeling our shift to an equity-minded approach where we don't punish ALL students for the bad choices of some? Are we willing to hold up a mirror to ourselves and examine why so many students are resorting to cheating to meet the demands of our program? Surely we can't say they are all bad apples! Are we considering solutions that emphasize the ethical values necessary to practice as healthcare professionals? What do our values on academic honesty and integrity look like? Have we continued to reinforce these values beyond just relaying them on the first day of orientation so that students can internalize their responsibilities as future healthcare professionals?

However, I started by voicing one question as I responded to my colleague's concerns, *"What is being done to understand what was driving the cheating beyond just the mere fact that assessments are always stressful to students and earning points is everything?"* Starting with this question is crucial to equity-minded assessments because it moves the focus from punishment to understanding root causes. This approach addresses equity gaps and student challenges by uncovering any systemic issues that are inhibiting a supportive learning environment.

Zero Tolerance Policies Diminish Moral Reasoning

In this situation, I chose to prioritize trust. Although most of my course director team wanted to implement zero-tolerance strategies and strict anti-cheating measures, I wanted to avoid creating an environment where students felt they were under constant surveillance and suspicion. It didn't sit well with me that if I wanted respect from my students, I couldn't extend the same level of respect to them. After all, I see my students as my evolving peers. Instead, I wanted to dedicate my energy to stressing the moral implications and the consequences for students who violate academic honesty. It seems more important to use this moment as a learning opportunity to articulate that academic integrity is key to our future as trustworthy healthcare professionals. My teaching philosophy holds trust as a cornerstone of my efforts, and I needed to share an honor code with my students in the name of transparency and mutual respect. In this case, I knew we already had provided lower-stake alternative assessment methods, but we didn't have a consistent dialogue running that stated that students have a responsibility to their own learning. When I presented my academic honesty oath to students on the first day of the quarter, I wanted to create a space for student discourse regarding disciplinary practices. While I can't change, nor wish to change, the University policies that were stressed on the first day of orientation, I did want to remind and empower students to hold themselves and each other accountable for their own learning.

Equitable Assessment + Competency-based Assessment = Fair Assessment

Equitable assessments ensure learners have an unbiased opportunity to demonstrate their competency. Ideally, we should also be giving our students multiple pathways to demonstrate their learning. Despite endorsing DEI principles, many educators might unintentionally perpetuate cultural assumptions or biases in their assessment methods, favoring objective quantitative approaches or only high-stakes exams. These methods often overlook the diverse experiences, cultures, and identities of students, reinforcing a deficit model for minoritized students. When disparities in Accreditation Council for Graduate Medical Education Milestones ratings for 2708 emergency medicine residents were retrospectively evaluated by sex and ethnoracial identity, it was observed that the underrepresented minority (URM) female residents consistently received lower ratings compared to the White male residents. These findings indicate a potential presence of intersectional discrimination in the evaluation of physician competency. Sex-specific ethnoracial disparities in resident assessments are emphasized as barriers to promoting equitable healthcare. By removing these barriers, there is a potential to enhance the retention and advancement of underrepresented trainees, ultimately fostering diversity and representation within the emergency physician workforce. Studies like this highlight that, unfortunately, many assessors overlook their own biases, resulting in flawed data and further marginalization of underserved trainees. Consider using your historical assessment data around student learning outcomes to discern effectiveness across different student populations.

Here are some other approaches you can adopt to have a more equity-minded perspective when designing your future assessments:

- Challenge assumptions about students' proficiency with technology, recognizing that not all students grew up with equal access or exposure.

- Support student success by providing resources such as glossaries for multi-language learners, ensuring equitable access to educational materials. Use terms that are accessible and familiar to a diverse student population.

- Start with the end in mind and play out "what if" scenarios to modify patient cases. What if the patient had financial limitations? Or developed a physical or cognitive disability? How would these factors change our approach to care or treatment?

- Patient cases are often written with a sense of deficiency that can perpetuate stereotypes (more to come on this in Chapter 22). Through which lens are we describing marginalized groups to our learners? What narratives are being constructed about a provider's responsibility to underresourced communities? It's essential to not promote we are saviors of patients; rather, patients grant us the opportunity to contribute to their care in partnership.

- Integrate the need to assess social determinants of health when patient cases are discussed to avoid pathologizing race or other identities.

- When scheduling assessments or post-exam reviews, consider all religious holidays and observances for timing of your exams and assessments (early during the day during Ramadan; avoiding exams after Sabbath starts, etc.). Proactively post religious holidays on your exam schedule.

- Utilize a team-based approach to provide peer review of assessments and any grading rubrics to minimize bias and lend diversity of perspectives. Include people who represent the cases you are writing (i.e., people with different abilities for a patient case involving a disability) to increase authenticity.

- Consider seeking feedback from students on the clarity of the criteria used in rubrics. Ask them to identify any areas of ambiguity or confusion that may impact their performance.

Overarching course design strategies that provide structure and promote well-being through the lens of assessments and grading include having clear expectations and grading policies that are communicated upfront. You can also provide timely and constructive feedback on assignments and evaluations and transparent grading criteria that give students multiple chances for feedback on their understanding and time to apply the feedback. For presentation-based assessments, I provide students with examples of what meets my criteria of excellence to help them visualize expectations and understand my standard of success. Try to minimize reliance on only high-stakes, end-of-term assessments as the main measure of performance and competency gain.

To ensure all students have an equitable chance at success, we must examine how our traditional assessment techniques might perpetuate inequities. Using post-assessment data has helped me in identifying and addressing disparities in outcomes among my students. For example, do certain demographics of students consistently fall below average exam scores in my course? How does their performance link to specific course learning outcomes? By disaggregating and analyzing our assessment data, we can also move closer to uncovering and addressing achievement gaps.

Key Takeaways

1. Instead of relying solely on punitive measures for academic misconduct, use a trust-based approach by emphasizing an honor code and fostering transparent communication about disciplinary practices.

2. Equitable assessments can offer unbiased opportunities for learners to demonstrate their competency while providing them with clear expectations, timely feedback, and transparent grading criteria.

3. To foster inclusivity in assessments, consider religious holidays, utilize team-based peer reviews to minimize bias, seek student feedback on grading criteria, and minimize reliance on high-stakes assessments.

CHAPTER 16

•

Facilitation Skills & Intergroup Dialogue

*"People fail to get along because they fear each other;
they fear each other because they don't know each other;
they don't know each other because they have not communicated
with each other."*
—Martin Luther King Jr

Intergroup dialogue (IGD), a face-to-face facilitated approach, is being used more readily across educational institutions and organizations. Developed in the 1980s at the University of Michigan–Ann Arbor, the goal of IGD is to foster active student engagement to gain deeper insights into social diversity and inequalities while also developing a sense of social responsibility. IGD was developed as a response to the growing need for educational methods that prepare students to navigate and lead in a complex, diverse, and stratified society—which is needed more than ever in healthcare. IGD is a structured social justice educational model that brings together individuals from different social identity groups to engage in open and constructive conversations about their experiences, perspectives, and social issues. It fosters a sense of community among participants and encourages collaboration and collective action, which can be harnessed to address complex DEI issues on a broader scale. This dialogue was originally developed for groups of 15-20 individuals with diverse social identities, but it can also be effective in smaller groups. The premise is based on the fact that interpersonal relations on campus are influenced by the historical and contemporary context of intergroup conflicts in the United States. In the health arena, this could be posing a discussion around how abortion bans can infringe on an individual's reproductive rights and limit their ability to make decisions about their own bodies and healthcare. Examining these conflicts through peer dialogues, rather than traditional 'banking' methods where educators act as experts depositing knowledge into passive students (see Chapter 10, "Students Aren't Objects of Learning"), fosters more active and transformative relationships and enhances interpersonal communication.

What key components are essential for effectively implementing facilitated dialogue in an online learning environment? The *Community of Inquiry* framework, based on research from Garrison, Anderson, and Archer in 2001, comprises three essential components: the need for the social presence of one another, in addition to teaching presence and cognitive presence. Their study found that group cohesion and a space for emotional expression are necessary to build a community of learning and inquiry, even in an asynchronous online course, despite students not being face-to-face in class. As more health professions programs are offering parts of their curriculum online, we see the continued need to be equity-minded in our course design.

Whether IGD is used in the classroom or experiential settings, it has often been reported to enhance participants' personal growth and increase self-awareness. I have personally been applying IGD in my courses for years. This approach not only invites students to share their circumstances but also trains them to actively listen to others—with the goal of reflecting on both our shared similarities and unique differences.

I have structured IGD around hot topics or controversial healthcare situations. For example, I have asked if students' individual Implicit Association Test results aligned with their explicit values. When discussing breakdowns in cross-cultural communication in healthcare settings, we have explored how our social identities can impact our ability to communicate effectively with patients. As we explore the attitudes patients or communities hold toward preventative health services or emergency services, I have used the Cycle of Socialization by Harro (see Chapter 5) to help students contextualize how social identities have influenced their own family's health behaviors. I recall a student sharing with her group, *"In my Filipino family, there is a strong emphasis to maintain a positive image of motherhood. Any signs of emotional struggle or depression are stigmatized. I've watched my own sisters and cousins be reluctant to discuss or seek help for their post-partum depression."* to which she was met with nods from various other group members who felt the same in their own cultural backgrounds. To take this dialogue to the next level, I posed to the group, *"What would be various strategies to reduce mental health stigma for each of your communities offered by a male versus a female practitioner?"* This created a space to foster a discussion about different approaches through their varying communities. Some students, particularly those who may feel stereotyped or belong to marginalized groups, prefer smaller and more supportive settings to express their thoughts and reflections.

As a facilitator, it was always important that I held space for student groups to debrief and unpack their emotions or reactions to each activity, while also grounding the exercise in establishing *group norms*. More to come on this in Chapter 17!

Chapter 16

Mastering the Art of Facilitation: A Vital Skill for Even the Seasoned Educator

I never fully appreciated the importance of facilitation skills when conducting intergroup student dialogue until I began to understand inclusive pedagogy. What I know now is that having effective facilitation skills is essential if we want to create safe and productive spaces for open discussion. Most educators and leaders would attest that having strong facilitation skills is a valuable trait, especially if one believes that discussion in our classrooms and clinical settings nurtures growth and learning. Yet, many educators don't receive formal training on facilitation skills.

In the spirit of cultural humility and life-long learning, even a seasoned facilitator engages in reflective practice, continuously evaluating and improving their facilitation techniques to create a conducive learning environment where IGD can occur effectively and respectfully. But far too often, we see two pitfalls: 1) educators take over the airtime and impart their own personal opinions, leaving little space for students to express theirs; or 2) facilitators maintain a neutral stance during the facilitation of student or trainee discussions, which by default allows for dominant narratives to persist. The reality is that in order to keep the IGD centered on the perspectives of students, we must monitor how much of our input we infuse during such conversations. Facilitators must actively listen to participants to understand their perspectives and emotions, which means *less talking and more listening*. Embrace silence. I personally had a hard time accepting dead air. I am a talker. However, I have seen firsthand how powerful silence is when we try to create safe containers for students to share. Silence is a space in time to pause and reflect, challenge our assumptions, process new learnings, and give others a chance to speak. *Don't be afraid of silence, embrace it.*

Furthermore, if we want to really lean into recognizing and honoring the differences across our learners, we must orient our lens to see past neutrality or impartiality and practice a more inclusive *multipartiality* approach when facilitating. We can't ask students to remove their sociocultural backgrounds and experiences from our learning environments. This request promotes what author bell hooks terms the "mind/body split," "where we ask individuals to compartmentalize and approach the classroom with a supposed objective mind." This would cause a disconnection from holistic learning.

Practicing multipartiality can help facilitators give equal consideration to multiple identities and experiences during these critical moments of learning. For example, teaching about the Belmont Act and the need for patient consent in clinical trials will address the origins of the Tuskegee Syphilis Study. Traditional teachings might present a sanitized version that overlooks the egregious ethical violations and harm inflicted on Black males in the study. Asking Black medical students to approach this history solely with an "objective mind" dismisses the intergenerational impact of such atrocities and the current mistrust of the healthcare system in many of their communities today. To foster inclusion and understanding, a multipartial approach would involve acknowledging and valuing the perspectives of Black medical students, recognizing the historical context, and incorporating a more comprehensive understanding of the Tuskegee Syphilis Study within the medical curriculum.

Multipartiality involves asking questions and challenging the status quo, not with the intention of persuading others to change their way of thinking but rather to recognize that there are multiple valid perspectives. When a colleague states, *"Students need to come to class to be successful on their boards,"* I might challenge this statement with, *"That's interesting. Where might you have learned that presentism always equates to academic success?"* Multipartiality is the practice of being aware of and acknowledging one's own biases and perspectives while also recognizing and valuing the perspectives of others, especially the counternarrative truths (see Chapter 5). There are other ways to be correct, and using this approach can help facilitate dialogue with students and colleagues because it encourages a more inclusive environment.

Multipartiality, as compared to holding a neutral stance, helps us also acknowledge biases and assumptions at play in the room while simultaneously recognizing the power we hold to drive the conversation as the instructor. We can use this power to limit any defensiveness or dismissiveness when we are faced with differing opinions or experiences. Disagreements and tensions are bound to happen during IGD, and facilitators need to address them constructively to keep dialogues productive. When we approach our facilitation through a multipartiality approach, we anchor to holding an open mind and a willingness to learn from others. We invite the varying perspectives and opinions into the conversation as participants. We push back against binaries that are "either/or" and instead encourage "both/and" in conversations. As facilitators, we must create opportunities for learners to share their unique experiences, particularly those who have been historically marginalized. For instance, I often ask in class, "Does anyone have different experiences from those shared?" This simple question opens the door for diverse voices and perspectives, amplifying the experiences of those who might otherwise feel overlooked. Ultimately, the goal of all dialogue is that it is productive, meaningful, and fosters mutual understanding and respect. Trust building is also crucial for IGD if we want participants to feel comfortable sharing sensitive or personal viewpoints, which enriches the inclusive environment we are aiming to build.

As facilitators of educational dialogue, we want to model that we value the differing perspectives of others while simultaneously creating an environment of inclusivity and belonging where we build community rather than create division. I have found this approach to cultivate collaboration, a greater sense of satisfaction in meetings, and engagement among all participants.

Key Takeaways:

1. Intergroup dialogue can foster deeper understanding of inequalities by allowing learners from different social identity groups to engage in open and constructive conversations.

2. Regardless of teaching experience or expertise, effective facilitation skills are vital for fostering productive and inclusive learning environments.

3. Practicing multipartiality helps acknowledge the diverse perspectives in the room while also addressing biases and assumptions to promote mutual respect and understanding.

CHAPTER 17

•

Support Through Restorative Justice

"I have a dream that we won't have to talk about 'restorative justice' because it will be understood that true justice is about restoration, and about transformation. I have a dream."
—Howard Zehr

Most educators desire to work within an education system that embodies integrity and harmony. However, the reality is that many of us commonly find ourselves encountering challenges like academic misconduct, breaches of conduct, and interpersonal conflicts among learners (and colleagues!). Unfortunately, these instances happen, and they are riddled with shame and blame. But what if we could have processes and practices to navigate these situations justly and with a focus on healing? *Restorative justice* originated as an Indigenous peacekeeping tradition and framework when harm needs to be addressed by multiple parties who have an investment in the event. In the educational setting, restorative justice is often linked to practices and policies related to academic misconduct. I find restorative justice to be important because it also has a proactive approach meant to foster community building. It can even be useful in cases of bullying, discrimination, or harassment. Ultimately, the goal is to prevent misconduct and conflict, promote fairness, foster compassion, and harness accountability so that a classroom or campus community can be anchored to a sense of trust. The added bonus is supporting the agency of individuals from disadvantaged communities.

One of the most prominent writers on restorative justice, Howard Zehr, defines the practice as "a process to involve, to the extent possible, those who have a stake in a specific offense and to collectively identify and address harms, needs, and obligations, in order to heal and put things as right as possible." Restorative strategies include both accountability and grace in a proactive and responsive approach. While restorative principles have been utilized in K-12 education for many years, they have yet to be fully embraced in higher education.

Restorative justice is a philosophical approach based on four principles: 1) inclusive decision making, 2) active accountability, 3) repairing harm, and 4) rebuilding trust. Karp describes restorative justice as one that "embraces community empowerment and participation, multipartial facilitation, active accountability, and social support. Another model that is often used is thinking of restorative justice as the "5 Rs" of *relationship, respect, responsibility, repair, and reintegration.* A central practice of restorative justice is a collaborative decision-making process that includes harmed parties, offenders, and others who are seeking to hold offenders accountable by having them "accept and acknowledge responsibility for their offenses; to the best of their ability, repair the harm they caused to harmed parties and the community; and work to rebuild trust by showing understanding of the harm, addressing personal issues, and building positive social connections." Restorative justice is not something we do to our learners, but rather, it is what we do *with* our learners.

Imagine you are a faculty member overseeing a dental clerkship, and you notice two of your dental students, Alex and Taylor, who seem to be having a challenge working together in the clinic. Their differing perspectives and interactions are causing tension. Alex privately approaches you to relay that he feels that Taylor is slacking and not taking the patient care responsibilities seriously, which he feels is impacting his ability to see patients effectively. You decide to use the restorative justice approach to address the situation in a way that promotes understanding and collaboration without creating a "victim" or "perpetrator" situation.

Gather Information:

Start by gathering information about the situation. Talk to Alex and Taylor individually to understand their perspectives.

Facilitate a Restorative Conversation:

Organize a restorative conversation involving Alex and Taylor. Create a brave space where they can share their viewpoints and experiences with each other.

Understanding Conflicts:

Help Alex and Taylor understand how their differing perspectives might be influencing their interactions. Encourage them to express their concerns openly and respectfully.

Address Concerns about Patient Care:

Acknowledge Alex's concerns about patient care. Discuss the importance of communication and teamwork in providing quality patient care. Encourage both Alex and Taylor to see the bigger picture as it relates to clinic workflow, responsibilities to quality patient care, and evaluation criterion of performance during their clerkship.

Chapter 17

Create a Collaborative Plan:

Collaborate with Alex and Taylor to create a plan for improving their working relationship. Discuss strategies for effective communication, cooperation, and setting clear expectations that value both students' needs and promotes effective teamwork.

Offer Support and Guidance:

Provide support and guidance to both students as they work on their collaboration. Offer advice on effective communication and problem-solving. Help Alex and Taylor understand how their ability to work together effectively contributes to better patient care outcomes and highlight the significance of their actions on the perception of the dental profession and on patient care.

Follow-Up and Reflection:

Schedule follow-up meetings to assess Alex's and Taylor's progress. Reflect on any improvements in their collaboration and address any ongoing challenges.

Building a community environment on campus and clinical rotations for healthcare students should be modeled on trust, closeness, respect, and dependability all around. This can be fostered by dedicating intentional time for daily discussions and open communication, especially when an incident that needs remedying arises. Restorative justice includes all stakeholders, provides equal time for everyone to share their input, and allows the instructor to serve as a mediator. Beyond sharing each person's facts of what happened, the harm and cause of the conflict should be addressed, and all parties should discuss acceptable outcomes or resolutions. As a mediator, I ask my learners to each share: *how they feel this problem should be fixed, how they would feel if they were the other person,* and *how they feel their behavior or actions could impact their peers.*

It is also important to address potential barriers to instituting restorative justice approaches. One is institutional culture, where there might be a prioritization for punitive measures, and it becomes a challenge to shift toward restorative practices. Furthermore, restorative justice pushes to empower all parties involved, which might run against the often-seen power imbalances and hierarchy between faculty, staff, and students in higher education. Given that restorative justice methods could require more time and trained personnel resourcing, some institutions may feel they are not ready or able to apply this approach. This does not preclude individual instructors from integrating restorative justice principles into their daily interactions with learners. However, if an institution wants to systemically embed restorative justice methods into its policies and culture, it is recommended to provide training for both educators and staff. Engaging in open discussions with students unfamiliar with restorative justice principles is also essential to foster a sense of accountability and community around the method.

Establishing Norms

As someone who has been raised in more of a collectivist tradition in my personal life, I have always felt a strong pull toward restorative justice because of its "we over I" spirit. This approach draws inspiration from the framework of a "community circle," where we can focus on creating a container of safety and partnership when shaping our classroom norms with our learners. Frequently, rules are dictated from a position of authority and do hold their significance, but inviting students to help create community guidelines for engagement helps them better engage in dialogues about the values we all share (e.g., respect, kindness, dignity, honesty, etc.). It enhances the harmony in our learning environments and peer relationships. Here are a few norms my students and I have co-constructed in my public health course:

- **Stay present, engaged, and relax your breath:** It is easy in our busy times to yield to distractions like our phones or laptops when the goal is to be actively listening to each other. Be mindful of your breath to stay present.

- **Audit your airtime during group discussions:** Ever noticed how some people can't resist jumping into the conversation while others hang back (shout-out to the introverts in the room!)? Let's face it, some people often dominate the airspace. But, here's the twist – recognizing our speaking time isn't just about fairness; it's about giving the quiet thinkers and deep reflectors their due time to think and share their perspectives.

- **Embrace the power of silence:** Picture this: the room falls silent during a challenging discussion. Awkward, right? But hold on! Silence isn't the enemy; it's the unsung hero of introspection and diving deep into fresh perspectives. Those quiet moments are also key to minimizing knee-jerk, biased responses, so we should embrace them.

- **Speak from personal experiences and not generalities:** Using "I" statements often takes more courage than "we" statements when we are sharing our thoughts or opinions. Rather than saying, *"We felt like the course was not fair because the exams were back to back."* Say, *"I felt like my work schedule was compromised because the exams were scheduled to close together."* This personal approach helps communicate your specific experience and concerns more effectively.

- **Lead with curiosity, not judgment:** Curiosity is healthy; it helps us grow and learn. But it is easy to have our implicit biases fire when we are listening to others' experiences, opinions, or ideas. We want to have an internal check when we find our judgments might be outpowering our curiosity.

- **We take what we learned; we leave who said it:** This honors the need to respect the confidentiality of what specific individuals say in our containers. It centers on trust building. For example, instead of reporting specific statements made by individuals, such as, *"Talynn, as an Asian woman, shared that she was called 'docile' and 'submissive' by her research mentor during undergrad,"* we rather share the collective insights gained, like, *"Our group found that microaggressions frequently occur in educational settings between educators and students."*

I would encourage you to think of other points that you could add to the "norms" of engagement that promote respectful dialogue in your learning environments. Invite your learners to add to them when you introduce them at the start of a course or group discussion.

Case Study: A Circle of Healing

In the aftermath of Hamas's attack on October 7, 2024, and the Israeli government's ground invasion of Gaza, a wave of contention swept through higher education institutions, sparking intense discussions, debates, and varied perspectives among students, faculty, and staff across the United States. As the faculty advisor for one of the largest student organizations on my campus with several Muslim and Arab members, I recognized the urgent need to provide a supportive space for students to process their emotions and navigate their collective grief. The enormity of the pain and suffering occurring in Gaza weighed heavily on the hearts and minds of many students who reached out to me individually. Students cried in my office, describing survivor's guilt and the

Chapter 17

inability to sleep or focus on anything school-related. I was right there with them. So alongside my student leaders, we co-created a series of restorative healing circles to engage in authentic dialogue, connection, and community building during a very challenging time.

A circle symbolizes inclusivity and unity. It is often rooted in ancient tradition and incorporates contemporary understandings about living in rapidly changing, multicultural societies. The Circle process, akin to the Arabic term "halaqa" meaning ring or circle, serves as an infinite container where empathy can be held for one another. It is a shape where decisions, dialogue, and belonging unfold, encouraging truth-telling without anyone being pushed to the sidelines. When we sit in a circle everyone can see each other. Learners can find a sanctuary to openly express their thoughts and feelings, and engage in communal recognition of grief, fostering a deep sense of relationship and safety.

Our circle sessions began with an exploration of the "why." I explained that we were holding these sessions to allow space to process our emotions, big or small, while being in community. We acknowledged the enormity of expecting normalcy in our daily lives amidst witnessing a genocide unfolding on our phones. The circle provided a reflective space to take deep breaths and just be. With no expectations or pressure to feel a certain way.

We also established the "how" of our circle by emphasizing our shared norms like listening with compassion, kindness, respect, and curiosity. We had to understand that each person present was healing and coping uniquely. Restorative circles are not about fixing anyone but rather creating an environment for personal narratives to be expressed. In this circle, our stories could be shared in confidence, and silence was embraced as an opportunity to connect with our inner guidance. We could take moments to pause and truly listen to what others were living through. We immersed ourselves in empathy, leaning deeply into understanding one another's experiences. We encouraged the use of "I" statements to honor individual processing and invited those who preferred not to speak but to just listen. We offered also for individuals to write down their thoughts anonymously as a means to release what was in the heart and mind space. We explored prompts like: What's one word that describes how you are feeling right now? What strength are you drawing on to get through this moment? What feels most important to your healing now?

Deep into the process of writing this book, a political or humanitarian resolution for the people of Gaza remained unresolved. Nevertheless, I noticed that facilitating several restorative healing circles for my students to navigate their intense emotions did prove to be beneficial. One of my Palestinian students expressed, "After attending the healing circle, I could breathe a little better knowing I was not alone in my sadness and frustration." It offered the students a sense of connection—easing their feelings of isolation, fostering self-care, and allowing them a space to process their pain and stress during a time of complex global tension.

Key Takeaways:

1. The four principles of restorative justice are inclusive decision-making, active accountability, repairing harm, and rebuilding trust.
2. Utilizing restorative justice, educators can facilitate productive conversations and collaborations among learners to resolve conflicts and improve teamwork in educational settings.

3. Restorative justice encourages the creation of inclusive classroom norms based on shared values, fostering respectful and supportive learning environments.
4. Restorative justice centers on grace, allowing for learning from mistakes, redemption, and the rebuilding of trust while also extending grace to educators for growth and progress in implementing these principles.

CHAPTER 18

•

Fostering Affirming Learning Spaces

"Prejudice is a burden that confuses the past, threatens the future, and renders the present inaccessible."
—Maya Angelou

Picture yourself trekking up the challenging terrain of the Rocky Mountains with a hefty 40 lb backpack on your shoulders. Your legs tremble with pain by the time you reach the 10-mile mark. Your lungs struggle for oxygen in the thin, high-altitude air. Finally, as you ascend the summit, expecting a moment of sweet relief, you encounter a group of people smiling, sipping coffee, and enjoying donuts as they take in the tree-top views. Glancing past them, you spot a food stand near the rest stop at your intended destination. One person remarks, *"Wow, you're so sweaty. Why didn't you just take the bus up here? Could have saved yourself the hassle."* Embarrassed and confused, your second look around reveals a service road with cars and buses making their way effortlessly to the summit parking lot.

Here's the reality of life: There will always be a service road with vehicles transporting people and their bags to the summit. While we all arrive at the same destination, some of us have to take the challenging path because we lack access to buses or even the fare

Chapter 18

for tickets. Some of us don't have the privilege of concealing our hike up the mountain and will arrive sweaty and tired. Some of us might attempt to mask our difficult journey by rushing to the restroom, wiping the sweat off our faces, and cleaning the mud off our shoes—anything to blend in and not be judged for taking the long way up.

Inclusivity and allyship demand that we don't assume there is a service road or that all our learners have a ticket for the bus ride to the summit of our programs. Making such assumptions widens the gap between us and our trainees, making it even more challenging to prioritize connection and create space for all students to be themselves. Culturally affirming spaces not only see but celebrate the differences we each hold—our journeys, our muddy shoes, and all. These spaces invite us to show and tell our whole stories. A psychologically safe learning environment recognizes that not every student has the same advantages and ensures that students feel secure, supported, and respected enough to freely express their thoughts, opinions, and ideas without fear of judgment or retaliation. In a psychologically safe classroom or clinical setting, learners are encouraged to take intellectual risks, engage in open dialogue, and share their diverse perspectives and experiences.

Talk Less, Listen More

"We are each other's harvest, we are each other's business, we are each other's magnitude and bond."—Gwendolyn Brooks

For several years, I have played an online game called "Spent" in my public health course of about 100 students to explore how social factors impact an individual's health status. The premise of the game revolves around the player experiencing a month of financial hardship. They must make tough decisions related to their health benefits, food, childcare, employment, transportation, and housing, with the goal of making it to the end of the game without losing everything. I break the class into groups of five students who must discuss their collective decision at each juncture of the game. I then ask students to write a personal reflective narrative about their experience working through the game in their groups.

Holding containers and space for people to share themselves is important and makes for a culturally affirming classroom. Here is one student's honest response that got me to sit and think about how I could better shift into integrating restorative practices in my course:

"When classmates laughed at the mom in the game for not being able to pay for her child to be in a sport, it felt like a knife in my chest. Then they laughed that they weren't going to let their kid have free and reduced lunches, and the more things they laughed at, the more the knife just got twisted and was dug deeper and deeper. I know that a lot of my classmates have parents that are doctors or they are more well off than my family ever was or is, and that's okay. But I know there's classmates like me that are going to be the first doctor[s] in their family [who] had free and reduced lunches. My parents came here the first time [and] they slept on a single mattress on a floor with nothing else. When my dad was deported, my mom followed, and then we found our way back. We all lived in someone's basement and I was a kid. I think that's the worst thing, I was a kid and I had the audacity to complain and not understand why my friends had big houses and yards and pools. I lived in a basement with no AC and I was obese because we couldn't afford healthy groceries and a whopper was 50 cents. Now [my mom's] a nail tech and cleaning lady and works from 8am-10pm most days and my dad from 12pm-3am. Two of my brothers were deported. One of my brothers was in jail for 4 years; I was in high school for the duration of that and then he was deported.

Chapter 18

I started working at 15 so I could stop asking my parents for money because my dad sent money to my family in Ukraine. My mom spent hers on me and mortgage for our condominium. If I had known just how expensive life was I wouldn't ask to be in sports or to go on school trips to Florida when my parents can't even get on a plane for fear of being deported. It's easy to assume that every student is rich and can afford to be at at this University. Truthfully, I can't afford to go to a private pharmacy school. Truthfully my mom couldn't afford to do everything that she did for me. She would starve so I wouldn't have to and that's the most beautiful thing that I hope I can give my kids one day. One day I know I will get my loans paid. One day me and my fiancé are going to buy a big house where my parents can live with us, not have to work and can rent out their condo so they can have income that doesn't involve barely seeing each other. Even though playing that activity in class was painful, I won't forget it. I know it'll make me stronger and better one day."

This student's submission made me pause. Later, I reached out to the student to acknowledge the distress in her submission and offered to meet one-on-one to support her through processing the difficult emotions. I then reflected on where I could improve, affirming each student's cultural identity while still providing a psychologically safe space to do so in my class. If I couldn't humanize the student experience during one interactive in-class game, then I couldn't really say I was cultivating an environment of belonging. If everything we do is transactional in the classroom or in our clinics, then we leave no room for relationship-building and mentoring. Both are essential elements for shaping a healthcare professional student's identity. It is not just about being sensitive to academic success but also having a willingness to understand how each person's identities and lived experiences bleed into the classroom.

You can't tell someone they belong, but you can make them feel it through cross-cultural interactions, conveying that "struggle is a part of life, but we can support you." If a student in a wheelchair with a disability has to think twice about attending an extracurricular event because they know the room will not accommodate their needs, that's a surefire way to say loud and clear, "You don't belong here." When a student's name is repeatedly mispronounced, or a transgender student's deadname is continuously used by an instructor, it clearly communicates, "You don't belong here." These moments push students further away from focusing on attaining the content we desperately want them to learn because they are too busy feeling anxious, worried, defeated, or isolated.

Here are a few ways to create culturally affirming spaces to cultivate belonging, foster psychological safety, and mentor our students more authentically:

- Hold time during class for counternarratives to be honored and engage in interpersonal dialogue so students can learn about one another and share cultural experiences.
- Model that differences and similarities in opinions and viewpoints can be honored simultaneously.
- Lean into our community norms to foster group discussions and ensure accountability. This is where restorative justice can also be exercised in Chapter 17. Embrace academic conflict as an opportunity to practice restorative justice, conflict resolution skills, and learning from crises.
- Engage in reflective, empathetic listening and emphasize the role of nonverbal communication (e.g., eye contact, facial expressions, yielding to technological distractions) to foster relationships.

- Ask students routinely to share how content intersects with their personal lives, academic goals, or community experiences.

Trauma Informed and Responsive Care

'Trauma is not what happens to you, it's what happens inside you as a result of what happened to you."—Gabor Maté

It is well known that a good amount of toxic stress is often seen as a rite of passage in healthcare training programs. The long work hours expected of medical residents, the intense pressure to manage high volumes of patients, and the expectation to stay updated on the latest evidence-based treatment plans are all too familiar. Regrettably, within the healthcare field, we often develop coping mechanisms to outwardly manage certain aspects of chronic stress. However, it's crucial to recognize that this stress has the potential to evolve into embodied trauma, manifesting as subsequent physical or mental health challenges in the future. As a mentor and preceptor, I have come to understand the significance of recognizing trauma in my students and residents. This understanding is a fundamental aspect of trauma-informed care. Whether we are students or educators working toward advancing equity and inclusion, we all bear lived experiences of trauma. This trauma may originate from historical, collective, or individual events in our past.

I have had the privilege of engaging in discussions with various institutions on how residency programs addressed the challenges faced by trainees providing care for patients during the COVID-19 pandemic from spring to winter 2020. There were a variety of differences in how trauma manifested. Programs that implemented regular check-ins and demonstrated empathy toward the negative emotions associated with working during the pandemic witnessed fewer instances of deeply internalized trauma among their house staff. Trauma comes into play, especially when it is compounded by a lack of or diminished coping mechanisms when stress demands increase. Trauma can show up as aggression, apathy, or even avoidance in our learners or workforce. When someone turns off their camera during an online course or seems disinterested while in class or on rounds, these moments serve as the pause moments that provide us with an opportunity to extend compassionate curiosity rather than judgmental assumptions.

Trauma-informed care, also known as trauma-responsive care, has gained increased attention in healthcare training programs in recent years. As educators, we have the choice to address and mitigate trauma within ourselves and adopt a curious stance toward understanding our learners' experiences. This involves broadening our perspective on others and creating an environment that allows our students to present their best selves.

To be genuinely trauma-responsive, it is crucial to be mindful of our most marginalized learners, recognize our role in mitigating stressful events, and work to minimize harm. An effective strategy is to provide students with a transparent *safety plan*—a set of tools or strategies they can rely on when they feel distressed during the learning process. For instance, at the beginning of class or rounds, you can share tools that help find calm, such as focused breathing, counting backward, visualizing a safe place with closed eyes, encouraging silent meditation or prayer, or even suggesting hand massages. If a student continues to feel overwhelmed, consider providing an exit strategy that respects and preserves their dignity and privacy.

To foster a culture change that moves toward healing and sustainability, it is essential to prioritize universal trauma responses

Chapter 18

and precautions. This shift will contribute to repairing and building a culture of resilience and ensure that our healthcare training programs prioritize the well-being of all learners.

The space between the occurrence of an event and our response to it is crucial. This space gives us the chance to make critical choices and learn. When we act impulsively without considering this space, we miss the opportunity to create inclusivity in our courses and a deep understanding of our learners. This space should make you want to reflect critically on how you want your students to express themselves, and how you can create environments that encourage all students without denying or ignoring their identities. This space also should make us want to explore the power dynamics that are often at play in academia, which compromise the opportunities for vulnerability to show up. For example, a Black student in a predominantly White institution or a queer-identifying student in a non-affirming learning environment might view being vulnerable or expressing their honest ideas as the opposite of psychological safety. Expressing ideas that might contradict the normative values of the society around them could seem threatening and compromise their grades or their chances for career advancement. So, if we are asking a student to be vulnerable, for example, through a reflective narrative or essay in the curriculum, this could threaten the psychological safety of our course. As an educator, it is crucial for me to acknowledge my power to alter these expectations for students and to respect their needs and boundaries.

Within the space between the event and my response lies an opportunity for me, as an educator, to challenge the existing norms and progress toward more equitable and inclusive practices. However, it necessitates a critical examination of how our power and privilege factor into the equation. When you make the choice to get more curious about the identities and experiences of your students, this gives you the leverage to use your power to create environments for them to thrive.

The current higher education system does not address the experience of being the only or the "other" in the classroom. For students historically marginalized, assimilation is often seen as the only path to success. For instance, a student may adopt a certain dress or hairstyle for access, to gain respect and opportunities in healthcare. The challenges faced by students with marginalized identities may not always be understood by their peers who are White, cisgender, Christian, or have other dominant social identities. Recognizing this is the first step toward creating a more accepting and diverse classroom that aligns with our professed commitment to inclusion in recruitment or retention efforts. Despite educators claiming to have their students' backs, it is essential to question if that's how students who are socially marginalized perceive their support.

Equity + Wellbeing + Inclusion = Student Success

A dear friend and colleague who was a racial equity champion in the UK once taught me her equation for designing a compassionate classroom, which I later added as a second step to my evolution to becoming an equity-minded educator. We must be willing to ask our students how, when, and where they learn at each stage of their academic journey. We must get curious about the barriers they face. Without the will to genuinely listen and believe their answers, we will continue to fall short of compassionate pedagogy. We must think about the students who are already feeling excluded and struggling and design our classes with them first in mind.

I routinely tell my students that they are always welcome to talk with me about any injustices they have personally experienced or stressors they may be facing outside of class. The least privileged students are most likely to be suffering from isolation; our Black and

Latine students, those with chronic illnesses or disabilities, those facing housing and food insecurity, or those who identify as queer. Our design for caring policies and compassionate pedagogy should prioritize them first, as we imagine how to promote well-being.

Several years into my teaching, I recognized the need to experiment with creating brave spaces for students to share their stories with me. I wanted to signal to students that they were experts on their own lives and how they wanted to be treated was paramount to my success as their teacher. I deployed a course survey asking questions like, "What do you wish teachers knew about you?" and "What do you wish teachers didn't assume about you?" I got responses ranging from "Just because I'm Asian doesn't mean I'm good at STEM," and "I'm proud of my accomplishments and status as a single Black mother; don't assume otherwise." When I asked, "What does inclusive learning look like to you?" students responded with, "It starts with a professor that makes me feel welcome, is positive, and really cares about my success despite my struggles or background," "A professor that has an awareness of all the inequalities among different races," and "[One who] makes us feel that class is a safe zone despite our differences and the different opinions we have." I've continued using these surveys to open the door for dialogue and to ensure that students' voices guide my approach to inclusivity. *Never take for granted what learners with marginalized identities share with you. Each time, they are often reopening their wounds to educate you.*

Case Study: What's in a Name?

Another simple yet powerful strategy to create spaces of belonging is to honor the sanctity of our given or chosen names. When we learn how to pronounce and write a student's, colleague's, or resident's name, we honor their identity. I recently shared a published commentary by two healthcare academics about the need to know students' names and strategies for pronunciation with colleagues at my college. I was met with an email looking for advice:

> *Hi Sally!*
>
> *I have been trying to be very cognizant of saying my students' names in class. Do you think it's better to potentially mispronounce the name but "try" and then ask for feedback (e.g., Did I pronounce that correctly?) or just not pronounce it at all and ask them how they pronounce their name (e.g., Could you please pronounce your name for me?)? I have heard both strategies suggested and wanted to get your feedback.*
>
> *My name gets mispronounced all the time, and I remember not correcting people as a student (and still sometimes today), so I understand the impact that this can have.*

And here was my response back:

> *Dear Dr. X:*
>
> *I totally hear you! For years I mispronounced my own last name to make it "easier" for colleagues and students but only recently realized I wasn't honoring my own identity ... names matter and are so personal, yes?*
>
> *I think showing the desire to be respectful goes such a long way when "trying" to say someone's name right!*
>
> *Of your two examples, the latter may go farther because you are acknowledging you want to get it right from the get-go...chances are that person has had their name mispronounced many times before, so it won't come as a shock that you are asking to hear it correctly right off the bat.*
>
> *Being proactive around names is also an important principle. For example, if I can proactively ask students to*

> *provide their names phonetically to me at the beginning of my class, it will give me a chance to practice saying them on my own time. It also shows that I care and that names are important.*
>
> *Hope this helps! Thanks for engaging with this content!*
>
> *In solidarity,*
> *Sally*

Honoring History

One of my first-generation Mexican-American students once told me, *"I connect best with teachers who have not been afraid to say the quiet things out loud."* When we often reveal sensitive or hidden parts of our history, this can leave an imprint of trust. One example of this I have done is by taking time to recognize and honor the ancestral history of the physical spaces we learn and work on by providing a land and labor acknowledgement. I often offer this at the beginning of a course I direct or a lecture I am invited to give. The acknowledgment focuses on the history, the present, and the contributions of Indigenous communities that we still reap the benefits of in our learning spaces.

Initially I felt unsure how to properly communicate the significance of recognizing the role that Indigenous and Native communities played on the land where my university and hospital stand. If this is the same for you, it is important to put aside the discomfort and shame. Instead, try to understand how colonial practices have contributed to present-day systemic inequalities. Reflect on the benefits that have been historically accrued across our education systems at the expense of marginalized communities. Investigating land acknowledgments has deepened my own understanding of the economic instability, lack of women's rights, and threats to children's safety caused by the trauma of colonization on Indigenous communities in North America. The interconnectedness of colonialism, environmental degradation, and medical science is explored in Rupa Marya and Raj Patel's book, *Inflamed: Deep Medicine and the Anatomy of Injustice*. They introduce the concept of "deep medicine," which I have used to teach my learners that illness, as presented in the body, should not be diagnosed only at the biomedical level. Instead, drawing on Indigenous wisdom, we should recognize that health is deeply intertwined with social and environmental well-being.

The concept of land and labor acknowledgment goes beyond recognizing historical injustices solely within the United States; it also serves as a symbolic gesture that we are mindful of ongoing oppression and occupations in our modern global context. This acknowledgment holds particular significance for our students who may have personal connections to regions with disputed land, such as Palestine, Western Sahara, and Ukraine. Students with ties to such regions see that, as an educator, I acknowledge the ongoing challenges faced by them, their families, and their communities—even if I don't have all the answers. This acknowledgment creates an opening for empathy and understanding, fostering an inclusive environment that recognizes the multifaceted impact of global conflicts on individuals within our educational community. It is a step toward building a community that values diverse perspectives and acknowledges the complex realities of students affected by conflicts worldwide.

Here is an example of a land and labor acknowledgment I present at the beginning of my course:

"We acknowledge that the land where we work and learn are the ancestral homelands of the people of the Council of Three Fires—the Ojibwe, Potawatomi, and Odawa—and many other tribes that resided on or migrated through the area for generations, including the Illinois, Menominee, Miami, Sauk,

Chapter 18

Fox, Kickapoo, Dakota, and Ho-Chunk nations. Our campus is also near an urban Native American community in Chicago and several tribes in the Midwest. The area was a site of trade, travel, gathering, and healing for more than a dozen other Native tribes and is still home to over 100,000 tribal members in the state of Illinois. We honor with gratitude the land itself and the Indigenous peoples who have been caretakers of the land throughout generations, past and present."

At the Crossroad between Disclosure and Self-advocacy

I have always believed that the path to becoming a healthcare provider is equal parts knowledge, empathy, and resilience. I have had the privilege of witnessing the dreams of countless learners take shape within the walls of lecture halls, simulation rooms, and hospital wards. With each of my learners comes a unique story, a distinct struggle, and an unwavering determination to make a difference in the world of healthcare.

One student I provided mentorship outside of class had an infectious enthusiasm for learning and an unyielding spirit to overcome challenges. He had cerebral palsy, a condition that left his right hand not fully functional, and he needed to rely on his left hand for most tasks. During his first clinical simulation, he was tasked with taking a medication history from a standardized patient and encountered an unexpected dilemma. He needed to take notes during the encounter to ensure he accurately captured every detail while displaying his ability to squarely face the patient and build rapport. However, his disability prevented him from holding a paper with his right hand while writing with his left. The solution seemed simple: resting the paper on the table beside him to find balance and stability. As the encounter concluded, the student found he had points deducted for not adhering to the standardized patient's expectation to face the patient—the paper that had provided him balance became a barrier to his success. Frustration and confusion swelled within him, leaving him pondering whether he should have disclosed his condition before the simulation began. I sensed his inner struggle and held space to listen as he expressed his disappointment following the experience. I gave him the opportunity to share ideas to solve such barriers... after all, our programs should nurture potential, not stifle it. Our candid conversation unearthed a hidden truth: the unwritten rules of healthcare education often leave learners at a crossroad between disclosure and self-advocacy. This student's story championed the notion that diversity of ability was a strength, not a limitation. The true measure of a pharmacy learner's potential lies not only in their medical knowledge but also in their ability to empathize, adapt, and advocate for both themselves and their patients.

When we think of disabilities, we can recognize that they are an integral part of our history, but learners and trainees with disabilities often face systemic obstacles in achieving their academic and healthcare goals. Physical and communication barriers, coupled with a significant lack of representation—evidenced by the fact that only 3.1% of physicians disclose disabilities—continue to be persistent issues.

It is time to break down these barriers and work toward an inclusive future where all individuals, regardless of ability, can excel in healthcare and education. This can start with operating from a *social model of disability,* where the responsibility is to make adjustments and accommodations so that individuals with disabilities can fully participate. For instance, if a student is hard of hearing, the program must provide clear masks in clinical care or an amplified stethoscope to ensure accessibility. This is very different from the often used medical model, which typically views disability as a deficit or a problem to be fixed or cured. It focuses on impairments and limitations and can perpetuate stigma.

Ableism further complicates matters, with stereotypes like "hearing is normal," "people in wheelchairs need constant assistance," or "someone with bipolar disorder can't hold down a demanding healthcare position" continuing to permeate our society. A multi-level ableist view operates on multiple levels. At the macro level, it includes physical barriers, policies, laws, and regulations that exclude individuals with disabilities. At the micro level, it manifests in social interactions, microaggressions, and social awkwardness, often resulting from ingrained biases. Furthermore, some students may hold internalized ableism, where they have internalized negative stereotypes or biases about their abilities, leading to a lack of self-confidence or self-advocacy. This is often why studies have found students with disabilities less likely to be forthcoming about their disability to their faculty or senior staff. Preceptors are often scared to open up this conversation because they don't know how to solve or support the learner once a disability or barrier is disclosed.

Creating an affirming environment means addressing any attitudinal or cultural barriers and knowing where to find resources when we are at a loss. Disability resource providers are important to identify so that they can determine accommodations for your practice or educational setting. We must break down the barriers for our students with disabilities, which means resourcing assistive technology like live captioning services, hearing loop systems, or even using AI-based speech-to-text software. At health centers, this could involve using options like teletypewriters, telephone systems with volume controls, language interpreter programs, and sign language classes for employees and teams.

Affirming Environments for Neurodivergent Learners

The term "neurodiversity," coined by Australian sociologist Judy Singer in the 1990s, encompasses individuals who experience a broad array of cognitive process differences, such as autism spectrum disorder (ASD), attention-deficit hyperactivity disorder (ADHD), and dyslexia. Embracing neurodiversity means accepting individuals for who they are and fostering an environment that allows them to thrive. If we want to reframe neurodivergence through a social justice lens, we must see this as a positive identity of difference, not one of deficit. We should understand that the lived experience of someone who is neurodiverse is often difficult, as they are living, working, and learning in environments that were not designed with them in mind. This reframing allows for recognition, celebration, acceptance, and keeping a positive outlook on disability.

The concept of neurotypicality, considered by many to be an illusion, is quite complex. While *The Diagnostic and Statistical Manual of Mental Disorders, Fifth Edition, Text Revision (DSM-5-TR)* acknowledges a spectrum of neurodiversity, defining where the spectrum begins and ends poses a challenging question. So then, what is neurotypical? Neurotypicality is often defined by the absence of certain behaviors or thoughts. In healthcare, neurodivergence is frequently positioned as a medical condition deviating from a biological norm, with the implication that intervention is necessary.

According to research released in 2023, 1 in 32 American children has been diagnosed with autism spectrum disorder (ASD). As a mother of a young child with ASD, I reflect on this statistic with a sense of wonder because I still live with the challenges of finding an inclusive educational space for my son's primary education. I have witnessed and grappled firsthand that non-affirming educational environments often stem from systemic issues, where certain expectations are imposed from the top down, leaving students to defend themselves. As a professor in higher education, I am also aware that many of my current students hold neurotypical passing privileges or remain undiagnosed, despite the growing incidence of ASD.

I have often observed neurodiverse learners mask their identity and needs in the classroom, leading to isolation and perpetuating stigma. A shift in perception is necessary. As I have gained insights into adult learners with neurodivergent diagnoses, a rejection of the medical model has become more apparent. This model can induce biases, as seen in qualitative studies where neurotypical individuals may overestimate their helpfulness, make quick negative evaluations, or not allow neurodivergent individuals the autonomy to express their strengths. Phrases like *"You should smile more"* or *"You don't seem neurodiverse to me"* can further contribute to the masking behavior, draining mental and physical energy in the attempt to be accepted. Acting "normal" not only leads to social exclusion but also compromises self-determination, self-efficacy, and self-care. Neurodiverse students desire social connections, but their behaviors may not align with neurotypical standards, leading to feelings of invalidation. It is crucial to emphasize that difference is not a deficit. According to the medical model, the framework of "fixing" individuals can hinder students from developing a positive self-identity and leveraging their unique skills.

As educators, we want our students to feel it is okay to be themselves. The neurodiversity movement is part of building an inclusive community that solicits and includes the voices of neurodiverse individuals. For example, the Autistic Self Advocacy Network's motto, "Nothing About Us Without Us," signals that people with ASD need to be involved whenever autism is discussed. This is really the essence of any affirming advocacy initiatives. For example, if your program is striving to integrate *universal design for learning (UDL)*, then engage your neurodiverse students in decision-making. UDL promotes flexibility and proactive approaches that promote a climate of inclusivity for all students. Here are strategies that could be used:

- Provide advance notice and clear instructions for class activities whenever possible.

- Consider the sensory environment (e.g., lighting, noise control, etc.) of clinical or educational spaces. Establish a confidential process for your trainees to communicate their preferences.

- Encourage movement and incorporate regular breaks to prevent the "dead eye" effect, where students look like they are disengaged. Access to nature for breaks never hurts!

- Communicate concepts iteratively, using multiple modalities (e.g., visual aids, videos, simulations, group discussions, etc.).

- Provide diverse options for completing assignments and demonstrating knowledge, recognizing that different paths can lead to the same learning objectives (e.g., infographics, written reports, oral presentation, video recording, concept maps, etc.).

- Establish systems for personalized care and networking (e.g., tutors, counselors, academic advisors, peer coaches, etc.) to build a community that ensures no student is left behind. Implement mechanisms to identify students in need and connect them with appropriate support.

- Foster safe spaces through supportive internal statements, anonymous surveys, focus groups, and caring conversations. Here's an example for your syllabus:

Neurotypicality is a myth. We all have different lived experiences, so our brains are different. These differences include both strengths and characteristics that empower us, as well as challenges to acknowledge, address, and work through. Our awareness of and identification with specific challenges, whether diagnosed or not, develops in our own time and way, and certain challenges may only become apparent during periods of high stress or effort, such as in graduate school. If you find yourself neglecting self-care/hygiene, struggling to sleep at night, missing meals, self-isolating, engaging in high-risk activities, having self/other-harm or suicidal ideations, or experiencing persistent emotional variability, please reach out. I will hold space for you and can discuss confidential, universally designed adaptations that may benefit your and your peers' learning. I can also make internal/external referrals for additional support services that are in line with your needs/preferences. I recognize and accept self-diagnosis of neurodivergent differences, as well as newly expressed, undiagnosed mental health conditions that may impact your academic experience. All information will be kept in confidence unless you provide consent to share or report having harmed or intent to harm yourself/others, which I am mandated to report for your and others' safety.

Building Affinity Spaces

Another avenue for creating a safe space and time for students who share a historically marginalized identity (race, sexual orientation, parental status, religion, age, veteran status, ability status, etc.) is to discuss shared concerns and support one another as they navigate their learning environments. Many students who hold marginalized identities don't have the confidence in their own identities to ask for what they need or to feel supported by the broader dominant group.

Affinity groups are formed with intention and defined purpose because here's the thing—we are tribal by nature. Despite our differences, we all yearn for a sense of community and true belonging where we are authentically seen, heard, and understood. We all seek spaces where we can show up as our authentic whole selves. For years, I struggled to express various aspects of my Iraqi-American identity. Despite the privileges I had due to the color of my skin and an easily pronounceable first name, I carried the invisible trauma of being a Muslim in a post-9/11 world, surrounded by xenophobia and Islamophobia. This left me feeling isolated, without a community that truly understood me. Little did I know that my own journey toward belonging and healing would intersect with that of some of my students who were searching for the same.

An Arab-American student walked into my office in 2012 looking for more than study advice. She came in looking for a connection and saw in me someone she could identify with. She relayed how her own community lacked health awareness and faced issues navigating the healthcare system. One I know from my own family's experiences. That conversation changed my trajectory when it came to teaching and mentoring my students. I realized that my students needed me to cultivate their potential by helping celebrate their identities; they needed hope that they could actively contribute to reshaping the narrative. Together, we could raise the collective to create meaningful and sustainable community work. What this experience showed me is that many students don't feel comfortable in themselves, especially based on their experiences that have been rooted in injustice and have pushed them to the margins of society.

Chapter 18

Creating affinity groups, whether through formal organizations or institutional efforts, provides a space where shared identities are celebrated. These groups not only empower members, but also help them achieve their goals in a system that often overlooks their needs. When students are given a space to gather and discuss how their school environments or training programs can be more equitable and meet them where they are, it can create strength to stand up for what is important that may not even be known to the administrators. For example, when a Jewish student group identifies that major assessments are being held on Yom Kippur, a Jewish holy day, the dates are shared with administrators to arrange accommodations for alternative testing dates. This ensures that no student faces stress or judgment for missing important assessments. Academic literature also supports that forming educational affinity groups is a powerful strategy for identity development and can enhance students' mental and physical well-being.

Obstacles are often presented as opportunities to learn and grow, but we must also ask when these obstacles become barriers to achievement. Disappointments are also par for the course, but we should be careful not to normalize them in healthcare education or allow them to become the most common narrative held by underrepresented students in health sciences. It is important not only to create psychological safety but also to recognize the need for psychological courage among students historically marginalized.

Here are a few guiding questions I encourage you to consider as you work on creating affirming and psychologically safe spaces in your educational setting:

- How do we attend to student differences, including social identities, background experience, physical and cognitive ability, and native languages?

- How can we deliberately foster classroom dynamics and pedagogical practices that effectively support the learning of all students?
- How can we leverage student diversity to maximize learning, including skills for working effectively with diverse peers?

Key Takeaways:

1. Prioritizing building compassionate relationships with students is more important for their learning than simply focusing on content delivery.

2. Inclusivity requires acknowledging that not all students have equal access to resources or privileges, and educators must be mindful of assumptions about their students' backgrounds.

3. Psychological safety is essential for students to feel comfortable expressing themselves and engaging fully in the learning process without retaliation.

4. Affinity groups can play a vital role in creating a safe space for students with shared identities, promoting identity development and overall well-being.

CHAPTER 19

•

Bias Intervention Techniques

> *"You can't eliminate [implicit] bias but you can 'learn how to dance with it' to minimize its effect."*
> —Howard Ross

A shift to acknowledge that biases, implicitly or explicitly, will always be a part of our world is not only key to the practice of allyship but also to eliminating systems of oppression in our healthcare settings and learning environments.

But what exactly is bias? Is it just stigmatized language in the medical chart—like dismissing a 36-year-old female's chest pain as mere reflux or anxiety, assuming that she couldn't possibly be having a heart attack? Or is it when a clinician uses tropes or slurs, such as believing that a patient's obesity is simply due to a lack of self-control, rather than considering the need for bariatric surgery? Or is it when we make assumptions about a learner's motivation based on our first impressions—like thinking an introverted resident who doesn't speak up during rounds is uninterested, instead of recognizing that she is also self-conscious about her accent? These examples from the literature illustrate how bias manifests in various ways, affecting our judgments and interactions. Bias can be defined as explicit or implicit inclinations for or against an individual or group. We have rules and laws to address explicit biases, ensuring accountability for overt discrimination. It's the implicit biases—the unconscious, ingrained associations we all carry—that require us to slow down and audit our thinking. All humans are neurobiologically primed to have implicit biases—they are always playing in the background of our minds. Think about who you perceive to be competent, professional, or successful... these perceptions are shaped by associations we have learned over our lifetimes. Variables such as our lived experiences, cultural backgrounds, race, socioeconomic status, religion, gender identity, and other aspects of our identities can significantly shape these ideas. What is more important than recognizing that we all hold biases is ensuring that we don't lead with them. Our snap judgments could undermine our ability to make sound clinical decisions, provide quality care, and build inclusive teams.

What makes bias even trickier is that, in some cases, it can be institutionalized or baked into our policies, practices, and structures. Dr. Elizabeth Chapman said, *"Cultural stereotypes may not be consciously endorsed, but their mere existence influences how information about an individual is processed and leads to unintended biases in decision-making, so-called 'implicit bias.'"* There are over 170 different types of cognitive biases that can easily influence our behaviors and decision-making in medical care. Public health advocate and physician Dr. Camara Jones describes the levels of racism and bias as born from cognitive or "mental shortcuts," where we recognize social patterns in healthcare and reinforce them with our behaviors. Vela and colleagues demonstrate this through their "vicious" and "virtuous" cycles of health. This model highlights the powerful interplay between interpersonal bias, determinants of health, the practice/learning environment, and provider decision-making.

Bias Intervention Techniques

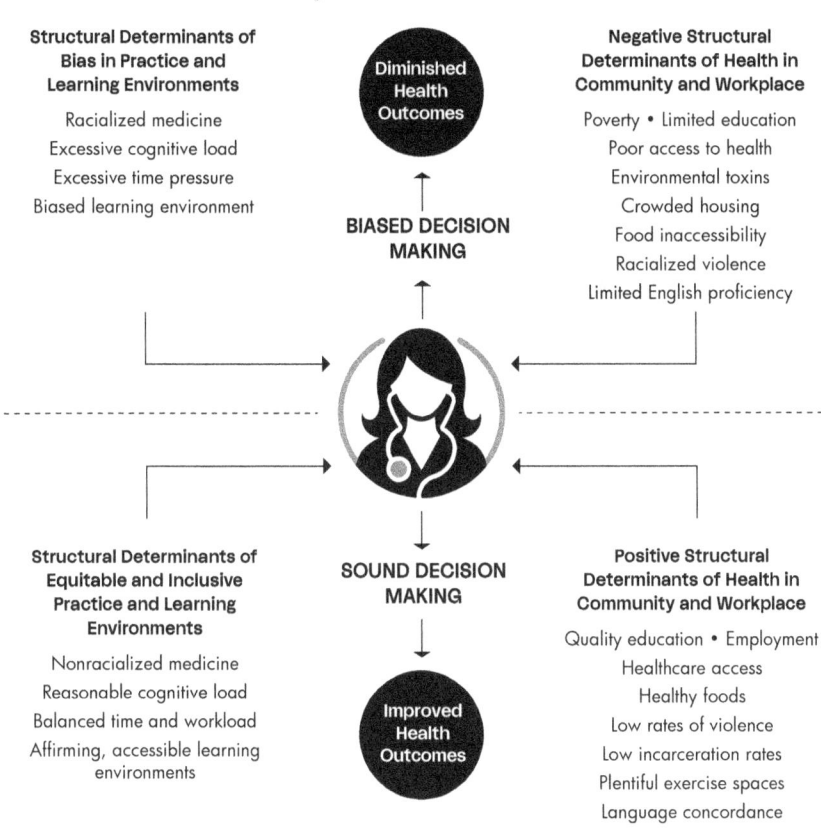

FIGURE 7: CYCLE OF INTERACTION BETWEEN STRUCTURAL DETERMINANTS AND PROVIDER BIAS

A vicious cycle is when we operate within biased practice and learning environments; we then make biased decisions that contribute to poor health outcomes. These outcomes are compounded by negative structural determinants of health in the community, reinforcing the provider's implicit biases. This is known as confirmation bias. On the flip side, in a virtuous cycle, we build

Chapter 19

more equitable and inclusive practice environments that can lead to sound decision-making to reduce health disparities and reinforce unbiased practices. These models can be helpful tools to discuss with our learners early in the training program. Our learners must enter practice with a clear understanding that denying the existence of biases or assuming immunity to them only perpetuates the harm they can manifest.

Microaggressions

In the 1970s, psychiatrist Chester M. Pierce introduced the term "microaggressions" as a way to describe the subtle insults and demeaning remarks that Black individuals routinely encounter. It was later expanded to include comments or actions toward any marginalized individual. Microaggressions are rooted in unconscious bias. Examples of microaggressions can span from asking, *"Where are you from?"* or statements like *"You speak good English,"* and *"I have Black friends,"* to *"Everyone can succeed if they just work hard."* It is not what is being said that is problematic, but rather, what the message is conveying. These comments communicate, *"You are different and don't belong."* While the intent might be a compliment or joke, the impact is that of harm. And let's be clear…there's really nothing "micro" about them. When these -isms happen, they can activate our nervous systems, and our body will respond with a whole range of emotions—from anger, worry, self-doubt, and shame to sadness.

In the healthcare training environment, the first step is to recognize when microaggressions are happening. It is when a Hispanic student is told, *"You are a credit to your people,"* or a Native American student is asked, *"You can educate others in your community about diabetes."* But what makes microaggressions so confusing is that they are not consciously delivered. They are powerful because they are often invisible to the person who made the statement, but incredibly destructive. Death by a thousand papercuts is often how microaggressions are described. Over time, the recipient accumulates the impact of numerous minor annoyances and insults, eventually leading to major consequences. Research has shown that healthcare professionals suffer mental health decline, depression, anxiety, and even physical health problems like allostatic loads from repeated microaggressions. Consequences also seen in studies include major medical errors and even suicidal ideation, which can't be taken lightly. For patients, this can manifest as lost trust in the healthcare system, dissatisfaction, non-adherence, and disengagement from their own care.

The social and cognitive impact of microaggressions can perpetuate stereotypes and cause us to devalue groups in our learning environments. Students may struggle academically when their energy is diverted from studying to managing the emotional toll of constant microaggressions. Students in health professions have reported losing focus on learning and training, feeling devalued and invisible, or even avoiding certain rotations and clinical sites because of historical encounters with biased patients passed down from one student to another.

I once had a female resident share feedback from her female advisor after a physician attending complained about her 'overly aggressive' tone. The resident admitted she had been passionate about advocating for her patient's pain management during medical rounds that day. Her advisor suggested, "My experience is that you'll get farther as a female working with men in this profession if you use a softer and more polite tone." Although the advisor meant well, her message reinforced a stereotype that women should communicate in a less assertive fashion. We can't make our learners think they need to "suck it up because this is part of the job." We must also acknowledge that we all have, at some point, been the source of microaggressions, and we need to shift our focus to repairing the situation instead of sitting on guilt, shame, and defensiveness when these situations are bound to happen.

Discussing topics like racism, sexism, and homophobia is inherently uncomfortable—most of us would rather talk about anything else. Yet, to cultivate brave spaces, we must normalize these discussions, including how to react when bias does occur. We also need to recognize that learners often struggle if they don't have a space to address bias safely during clinical care. In many aspects of healthcare training, the roles of learner and teacher are well-defined. However, when it comes to bias intervention, the clinical hierarchy must be challenged. A medical intern might better understand how to handle bias than a seasoned provider—so don't be afraid to ask learners for their ideas. Creating an inclusive atmosphere where everyone feels welcome to share and contribute is a prime element of bias intervention training. For instance, some institutions have implemented 'DEI Rounds' or 'DEI at the Bedside' curricula to facilitate intentional team-based discussions about bias—how it shows up and what impact it has on patient encounters or healthcare team members. These models address knowledge and behavioral gaps, and provide learners at every stage of training with language they can use in real-time within an existing inpatient clinical rounding infrastructure.

Bias Awareness and Accountability

Bias is hardwired into our brains—there's no escaping it. Everyone has likes and dislikes, and this isn't necessarily a bad thing. But it becomes problematic when we fail to recognize that our biases can be an obstacle to inclusion. If we don't step up and take responsibility to interrupt them, we risk allowing them to quietly erode our relationships and decisions. Educating our learners on the different types of bias, how they show up, and what to do as an upstander and patient advocate is essential.

Each year, I have my pharmacy students write a reflection about bias, following an interactive in-class activity called "Trading Places." The goal is for each student to better understand how their biases are rooted in stereotypes about different identities. During this activity, students are presented with a description of 10 different individuals from different professions, ages, races, ethnicities, abilities, and so on. They are then individually asked to rank who they would trade places with for one year from the list and why. One first-year student wrote about how the activity linked to her past experiences and future role as a healthcare provider:

"Being a patient advocate means calling out inappropriate and or racist behavior whenever we see it, but especially in the healthcare setting. Throughout my life, I have rarely seen outwardly explicit racist comments; I've more commonly seen and experienced microaggressions. If people are being obnoxiously racist, those instances are typically easier to call out. The harder ones are the microaggressions. In high school, one of my best friends, who is Black, took out her braids and wore her natural hair. In class one day, someone said to her, 'Hey, your hair is a lot bigger today.' They didn't say it as a compliment, but she responded, 'Thank you' anyway, and smiled. The comment made me uncomfortable, but I wasn't sure what to do. I talked to her about it later, and she told me, 'It isn't worth the hassle.' I left it at that, and I wish I hadn't. Advocating in the healthcare setting is so important because I wouldn't ever want a patient to have the mentality of, 'My health and my well-being aren't worth the hassle.' My friend's passive attitude toward the situation made me sad, but I wasn't sure how to be better or make the situation better in high school. I've learned through this class that simply speaking up and drawing

attention to the issue is a start, and it makes a world of a difference to the patient/person, so they know they're being heard and they're worth standing up for. I think it's important to understand you might not change people's minds with one conversation, but there are things you can do to make a situation right. And advocating on behalf of patients is the bare minimum we can do to honor the oath we take to serve our patients with dignity and respect."

You don't have to look too hard to spot bias. Let's consider the use of stigmatizing language in the electronic health record as just one example. Many clinicians are used to seeing negative descriptors like "challenging," "non-compliant," "defensive," and "agitated," which are more often associated with minoritized patients. This is backed by a recent study by Sun and colleagues that used machine learning to analyze over 40,000 electronic health records, revealing that Black patients had 2.5 times higher odds of being labeled with at least one negative descriptor compared to White patients. We also see this with studies that show that stronger provider bias is associated with poorer patient-provider communication. For example, physician bias is shown to influence talk time with patients, including interruptions.

How do we do something about addressing implicit bias? Beyond individual accountability, as an institution, we need to measure the impact of bias and not just the intent of avoiding it. We also need to engage our clinical staff, learners, and faculty in bias intervention training to minimize the impact bias can have on the delivery of quality healthcare.

A small note as someone who has designed and delivered numerous bias training programs or modules (including those for continuing medical education credit)—while these programs are great at providing the foundational language and raising implicit bias awareness, relying on them alone will not eliminate bias in individuals or workplace environments. They often don't have follow-up, nor do they necessarily change behaviors sustainably. Training programs must encourage actionable and comprehensive institutional change strategies to root out the causes of biases in our structures, policies, and procedures.

Breaking Bias: Responding with Impact

Confronting biased and offensive language or behavior requires courage. And I promise you, the first time you address a bias, it will be nerve-wracking. But, just like anything else, practice affords us the opportunity to build confidence and skill. Two principles are essential when interrupting bias as a bystander: 1) focus on the person harmed and ensure their safety; 2) consider how and when you want to intervene. Let's start with the first, where we confirm the safety and comfort of the person who is the recipient of bias. We have to validate their experiences and feelings in the moment or soon after through statements like, *"That was not okay what happened there,"* and then ask how you can assist them with a question like, *"How can I support you?"* or *"If this happens again, how would you like me to respond?"* Don't assume you know how support might look. Maybe they don't want you speaking on their behalf. Maybe they have specific expectations about how they would like you to show up as an ally.

Next, consider if this is the *time* and *place* to really address the situation. If it is, then think about the best strategy for interrupting the interaction. Again, our goal is to always preserve the dignity of all individuals in the situation. Most models start with *noticing the event*. You can't assist when you don't see it. I like to use the PAN acronym: Pay Attention Now. Just like a movie camera "pans" an environment to show the whole picture, we need to continuously PAN our environment to notice patterns of treatment. We should pay attention to behaviors, comments, and feelings to be objective and avoid falling into a snap judgment or creating a "story" about what we *might be* seeing. We should also notice the identities of the people involved to better interpret and add context to the situation.

Researchers Kupiri Ackerman-Barger and Negar Nicole Jacobs have developed the roles of microaggression scenarios and the "Bystander-ARISE Approach," which can be used to investigate how we can intervene:

A: Awareness of the microaggression (again, think PAN)

R: Respond with empathy (avoid judgment)

I: Inquiry of facts (ask, "What did you mean by that?")

S: Statements that start with "I" (talk about how it made *you* feel)

E: Educate and Engage (Fill in the gaps of what was intended vs. the impact of the person's statement. This might sound like, "I know you didn't intend to stereotype people with disabilities, but as your colleague I wanted to share with you how it came across that way.")

Another model that can be used for bias intervention is the *4D Model: Direct, Delay, Delegate, Distract*. These D's can be used in combination if needed.

Direct: This approach involves directly confronting the person who made the statement and assertively addressing the harm caused. Example: *"Hey, I overheard your conversation. It sounds like you are feeling worried or scared about someone using the 'wrong bathroom.' I thought it might be helpful for you to know that the university has made it clear that everyone has the right to use the bathroom that fits their identity; they even released a policy statement about it that I am happy to share with you via email."*

Whether addressing a colleague at work, your student, or a person in your personal life, *link to commonly held values or norms.* This will disarm the situation, reduce any defensiveness, and tend to be more effective before addressing the behavior or biased statement. Direct approaches can take the form of either *calling out* or *calling in*:

- "Calling out" sounds like *"I know you are dedicated to our hospital's stance on inclusion and creating a positive work environment. It is crucial to uphold these values by ensuring that no one feels excluded or unwelcome due to their identity. Yesterday, I noticed our colleague Ahmed felt singled out as a Muslim when you assumed everyone was celebrating Christmas and would want to contribute to the holiday party."*
- "Calling in" sounds the same, except you come from a place of inquiry like, *"I'm curious why you think everyone on our team celebrates Christmas or wants to contribute to the holiday party?"* Coined by scholar-activist Dr. Loretta Ross, this approach allows the person to pause and discover their own assumptions. You can follow with, *"I'm curious if this could make our colleagues like Ahmed feel othered as a Muslim."* or *"I noticed Ahmed seemed uncomfortable when you mentioned the Christmas celebration yesterday."*

Delegate: Scan the situation and determine if there might be a risk to intervene yourself and delegate to a third party who might be better positioned to assist. This could be a direct supervisor, equity officer, Department chair, or Title IX officer.

Delay: Sometimes, we need a minute (or longer) to formulate our response to a witnessed bias. Delay is a step that can buy time or even be used to follow a direct approach, in which you check in with the recipient of the microaggression to address the hurt. Delay also gives us time to educate ourselves about the next steps to take to be in solidarity with the person harmed. Delays can also be seen as a speedbump to slow the conversation by saying something like "Ouch!" or "Whoa! I'm not sure that sounds okay to me. I need to process that." I often tell people to not be afraid to disengage if things get too heated or emotional in the moment.

Distract: In the moment, we may not know the best way to directly intervene, so de-escalation of the situation by distracting attention away from the person being harmed can help. This should still be followed by checking in the recipient of bias. Some examples of distraction tactics include asking for the time, moving to the next agenda item during a meeting, asking an unrelated question, or even spilling your drink.

Navigating Patient Bias and Microaggressions

In the realm of healthcare, we must also talk about what to do when a patient displays biased or discriminatory behavior. Recent survey studies have shown that 47% of physicians, 34% of registered nurses, and 44% of nurse practitioners report bias-based reassignment requests. Additionally, 59% of physicians and half of registered nurses and nurse practitioners have faced general identity-based bias, with Black and Asian physicians experiencing the highest levels of such bias. Often these go unreported in medical settings so as not to disturb the code of "professionalism," especially by providers who carry marginalized identities.

I still vividly recall the first time I witnessed an older male patient tell my Asian student on her internal medicine rotation at the Veterans Affairs hospital, *"You have good English for a Chinese person,"* after she introduced herself to take a medication history. My student was not Chinese, and she was born in the United States to

Korean immigrant parents. I watched as she showed shock, then smiled awkwardly, looked down at the floor, and shyly said, "*Um, thank you.*" As a preceptor witnessing my student's struggle with how to correct the patient, I knew I had a duty to intervene and practice my allyship. I stepped in to correct the patient's biased comment, shielding my student from further interaction with someone who may have meant well but had inadvertently caused harm.

Beyond being awkward, these situations have an ethical component to them, especially when learners are at risk to microaggressions or bias because of the power dynamics at play in the healthcare setting. Students are most vulnerable because they often lack the knowledge to handle such situations and have limited decision making authority. Furthermore, there is also a concern that they may be perceived as flawed or face academic repercussions.

The ethical dilemma faced by healthcare professionals and educators is the implicit expectation to care for patients, irrespective of their behavior. While this commitment to patient care is paramount, it is equally essential for learners and clinicians to be treated with dignity and respect in the workplace. These issues start early and continue throughout our practice. This discussion requires us to start by defining how patient bias can show up. It can include incidents like explicit rejection of care, prejudiced epithets, inappropriate compliments, flirtatious comments, and belittling jokes reflecting racial or gender stereotypes. Recognizing and addressing these manifestations is crucial not only for the well-being of healthcare professionals but also for maintaining a healthcare environment that upholds the principles of equality, respect, and inclusivity. Balancing the duty to care for patients with the need to establish and maintain a respectful workplace is an ongoing challenge that necessitates us to have open dialogue and proactive strategies for addressing bias in our healthcare settings.

Chapter 19

Case Study: Supporting Learners Experiencing Incidents of Patient Bias and Discrimination

Imagine you are precepting a female Black nursing student who is checking the vitals of a White male patient on the general medicine floor. The patient calls the student "colored girl" three times in front of you. You notice the student doesn't respond but visibly seems uncomfortable. How would you apply the 4Ds (Direct, Delay, Delegate, Distract) to handle this situation? How would you respond to the student? Or to the patient?

Being proactive is key to advocating and taking responsibility for your learners while on rotation. If we don't speak up or respond, we can inadvertently send a signal that we condone this behavior from patients and perpetuate the systems of discrimination that exist more often than we wish.

When you first meet your learners, set expectations and discuss protocols for responding to biased patients. Remember to also discuss when a student or resident might wish to handle a situation independently. If you think a patient's comment is making a learner feel disrespected or devalued, consider speaking up. It is not the medical students' responsibility to advocate for themselves! After the incident, debrief with the student. Give them an opportunity to talk about what happened without minimizing their experience. Guide them in crafting an appropriate response if a similar situation happens in the future.

During my orientation with rotation students at the hospital, I set expectations by saying, *"There are times when a patient may say something that is disrespectful or derogatory to you. Though rare, they do occur. You can absolutely step away from any experience that makes you uncomfortable. I am here to be your advocate. Let's talk about how you might respond in these situations if they occur and what resources are available to you."* When you witness bias from

Bias Intervention Techniques

patients toward students, you can intervene at the moment by saying to the patient, *"We don't think you meant to be hurtful, but your comments are making us feel uncomfortable. We promise to treat you with respect, and we expect the same from you."* Learners appreciate when these incidents are addressed at the moment when possible, and debriefing afterward is always helpful.

We also need to integrate debriefing with the student, regardless of which 4D approach is used, by starting the conversation with something like, *"I'm sorry, that should never have happened,"* or *"How are you feeling? How can I best support you right now?"*

On a systemic level, bias in healthcare institutions and learning environments must also be addressed in order to promote a culture that centers on reporting and respect for clinicians. Patient satisfaction is an important metric for health systems, but this should not deter us from creating guidelines for patient conduct and clear policies to protect clinicians and provide reporting mechanisms. As early as pre-experiential learning, we need to educate our learners on their rights and responsibilities. For our preceptors, we need to provide support and training on how to respond in these situations. I have found that serving as a mediator is also helpful. It can just be the tip of the iceberg when we see an issue with bias surfacing in the classroom or in our healthcare settings. Facilitating dialogue requires expertise to avoid creating more harm. Don't be afraid to bring in outside experts on inclusion, community building, and equity to help the team and organization through the murky waters.

"I had to deal with another patient telling me to go back to my country at the pharmacy. I can't keep going to work with this level of Islamophobic rhetoric. I just don't feel safe." These are the words of a female Muslim student who wore a hijab and had dealt with several incidents of patients saying racialized and anti-Muslim statements

to her with very little support from her supervising pharmacist. My first thought was to ask about the patient code of conduct policy at her pharmacy. Despite clinicians doing their best to deliver the highest quality of care to patients, there can still be harm caused by our patients; all healthcare professionals must understand their rights, while patients should have clarity on what is unacceptable. It is okay to be completely shocked by a patient's comments or need the time to process your emotions in order to respond appropriately. Many healthcare systems have started to display and communicate a code of patient conduct in their settings. These codes should also be shared with trainees as they learn their rights to practice in a safe and caring environment. Patient conduct rules could include:

- **Respectful behavior:** Patients must treat clinicians with respect and dignity, recognizing their expertise and dedication to providing quality care.

- **Non-discrimination:** Patients must not discriminate against clinicians based on their race, gender, ethnicity, religion, sexual orientation, or any other protected characteristic.

- **Personal boundaries:** Patients must respect the personal and professional boundaries of clinicians, refraining from any behavior that may be considered intrusive or inappropriate, including physical or verbal threats or assaults.

- **Verbal communication:** Patients should use respectful and appropriate language when communicating with clinicians, avoiding any form of verbal abuse, vulgar language, threats, or derogatory remarks.

Recovering from Missteps

> *"The best apologies are short, and don't go on to include explanations that run the risk of undoing them."*
> —Dr. Harriet Lerner

As long as we are imperfect humans, mistakes will happen. It doesn't matter if you are an expert on all strategies of bias intervention; expect to still mess up. More important than the mistake is how we recover and practice cultural humility. This means we put aside our ego, acknowledge our error for what it is, and take responsibility for the impact of our mistake.

Leaning into the principle of *impact over intent* (see Chapter 11) means we recognize the consequences of our missteps and take a pledge to do better next time. When this happens, here are other steps to take:

- Apologize and take responsibility for the mistake.
- Ask how you can support the person affected going forward. Their idea of support may look different than yours.
- Engage in self-reflection and acquire additional knowledge if needed.
- Avoid justifying your intentions. When we say, "I didn't mean it that way," we undermine our apology.
- Do not expect instant forgiveness or appreciation (they may need space and time to process).
- Do not disengage or cease your efforts to keep learning.

Chapter 19

Now, it is your turn to see how you would intervene when a bias presents. Take a read of each scenario below and describe 1) Your initial reaction. 2) Which of the 4D's might you employ besides the "direct" approach? 3) How can you use the practice of *calling in* to initiate a constructive conversation and advocate for the learner?

Scenario 1: You hear your colleague mispronounce the name of a new medical intern, to which the resident responds by correcting them with the right pronunciation. Your colleague then says, *"Sorry, your name is like 15 letters long. I'll never learn how to say it right."*

Scenario 2: Your colleague notices that a student listed their hometown on their admission paperwork as Mexico City, Mexico. They make the comment to you, *"It must have been so hard to grow up in Mexico with all that poverty. They are so blessed to have moved to the US!"*

Scenario 3: You're a clinical pharmacist on medical rounds. A new, Black female medical intern on your team presents her patient case. The attending physician with whom you have worked for several years responds, "Wow, you're so articulate, great job!" You notice the intern not smiling and looking down embarrassed.

Scenario 4: A student is talking to a clinical instructor about their academic struggles as a first-generation student. You hear the instructor respond with, *"I had struggles, too; it has nothing to do with being a first-generation graduate student."*

Bias Incident Reporting Systems

Incidents of bullying, harassment, and hate have unfortunately become more prevalent in an ever-polarizing world. Campuses and healthcare institutions are not immune to these challenges. Acts of discrimination are inevitable. At the very least, we need a shared understanding of how our institutions define bias so we can recognize it when it occurs. Furthermore, we must be willing to speak up about bias if we want to see the negative effects minimized.

A commitment to action around bias is demonstrated by having a reporting system in place. Reporting is important to show accountability to addressing bias incidents that compromise inclusive environments. But why don't individuals want to report when a system is available? Often, "It's a personal" or "confidential" situation is used as a guise for a lack of dialogue or accountability when bias occurs. I have often heard faculty and learners express frustration with institutions being disingenuous—encouraging people to report incidents of bias but failing to act on it when they do erodes trust and discourages future reporting.

We must acknowledge the power dynamics in place when reporting systems and policies are created. A learner who is already minoritized may often feel a risk when reporting an attending or a professor for bias or harassment. Similarly, a junior faculty member may feel their promotion or tenure could be jeopardized if their report is mishandled. Often, those reporting want to understand who is receiving their report on the other end. While this role could be held by various members of the university or health institution, it is critical that these individuals are extensively trained on the institution's culture, bias and microaggression intervention strategies, and conflict resolution using restorative and transformative practice.

In order to take meaningful and sustainable action to address prejudices and bias in a healthcare or higher education institution, bias reporting and response processes should be built into the strategic plan for the institution at large. The structure of an easily accessible and responsive reporting system is important and should follow two main principles:

- It should support the person/community impacted by the act of bias/prejudice and center the concerns and desires of those who reported the bias. From a restorative justice practice, they should be allowed to share how they would like to see justice achieved and be part of the plan for resolution of the situation. For example, if a learner reports microaggressive comments from a peer during a clinical skills lab, they should have the chance to suggest what resolution would look like for them. The responders should integrate this into the plan.

- It should be relayed to those who report a bias that if they include their contact information, they will be protected as an individual from retaliation and be offered a confidential meeting to discuss the incident and be offered information about related institutional policies, procedures, and resources. A mechanism for reporting and remediating discriminatory incidents without risk of retribution is essential. Within higher education, Family Educational Rights and Privacy Act (FERPA) regulations should be adhered to when handling reports and information submitted via a campus online portal.

As we collect data on incidents of bias, it is best practice to continuously evaluate it to identify trends and understand the challenges faced by our institutions. This can inform updates to our policies, educational programs, and administrative actions.

Key Takeaways:

1. While no one is immune to implicit biases, recognizing them is vital for allyship and dismantling oppressive systems in healthcare.

2. Microaggressions, often invisible yet impactful, can harm mental health, perpetuate stereotypes, and create cognitive loads for learners in healthcare professions.

3. Combating bias requires proactive measures such as promoting awareness, holding individuals and institutions accountable, and fostering a reporting culture in healthcare and learning environments.

CHAPTER 20

•

"Cultural Competence" in the Curriculum

"When 'I' is replaced by 'WE,' even ILLNESS becomes WELLNESS!"
—Malcolm X

The importance of cultural humility was stressed as we discussed "the principles" in Part 2 of this book. What I didn't elaborate fully on is that practicing and role-modeling cultural humility is a dynamic, lifelong process. It requires deepening self-awareness, openness, and ongoing learning. One that requires a more nuanced and respectful understanding of diverse individuals and communities. Within health education, cultural humility has quickly been replacing educational standards that still work off a model of *cultural competence,* which implies a fixed set of knowledge and skills, potentially leading to stereotyping and bias. While my preference is for the cultural humility model, for the sake of connecting to the currently used lexicon, I will use "cultural competence" or "cultural competency" in this chapter.

Most healthcare professionals can agree that a core tenet of our work is to promote and advocate for equitable and positive health outcomes for patients, regardless of their cultural background, race, ethnicity, sexual orientation, or other facets of social identity.

According to the Association of American Medical Colleges (AAMC), there are multiple processes required to eliminate racial and ethnic disparities in healthcare, with education cited as the primary method to develop culturally competent physicians. Often, we operationalize our educational standards in our programs so our learners integrate a "patient-centered" approach to care, where patients are partners and active participants in their treatment plans. But what if we elevated our cases and teachings to integrate a more holistic and broader *"person-centered" or "people-centered"* approach to care?

Endorsed by the World Health Organization (WHO) and various global bodies, person-centered care emphasizes that a patient should not be solely defined by their illness or diagnosis. Instead, it embraces a more inclusive perspective that considers the broader context of health, which includes family, communities, and society. Rooted in the principles of human rights, dignity, autonomy, empowerment, and well-being, person-centered care recognizes the multifaceted nature of an individual's health.

A person-centered approach goes beyond just biomedical factors and allows for a more comprehensive understanding of how health is influenced by the larger context of health policy and health services. This relates to the concept of *structural competency*, which moves beyond an individual-level view of cultural competence to explore how social, economic, and political structures influence health inequities and healthcare delivery. These factors can present as symptoms and conditions like depression, substance use disorders, hypertension, diabetes, and trauma.

When educating our trainees, it is beneficial to adopt a wider and more holistic perspective in explaining patient care. This

"Cultural Competence" in the Curriculum

approach facilitates the integration of health equity measures and the exploration of structural factors that impact patient care, advocacy, and the potential improvement of the healthcare system.

Integrating health equity and disparity content into academic pedagogies of health professional education, including medical, nursing, and pharmacy education, is not a recent calling. We understand that disparities continue to persist across most areas of disease states and illnesses we are trained to manage. As I write this book, it has been over 20 years since the Institute of Medicines (IOM) recommended integrating cultural competency into the curricula for all healthcare professional students in its 2001 report, *Unequal Treatment: Confronting Racial & Ethnic Disparities in Healthcare*. This was a strategy to address racial and ethnic disparities due to lack of access, which the IOM attributed to possible bias, stereotyping, prejudice, and uncertainty among healthcare providers in caring for patients from diverse backgrounds. A systematic review of the effect of cultural competency in healthcare settings shows evidence of positive effects on patient health outcomes and access to care.

Evaluate the Depth and Structure of Your Cultural Competence Content

If our ultimate aim as healthcare educators is to develop compassionate practitioners who can serve a diverse patient population, we need to invest in cultural competence curricula. This means that we stress within our teaching the importance of holistic patient assessment, the appropriate use of patient demographics (e.g., race, ethnicity, socioeconomic class, gender, etc.), and highlight the influence of healthcare beliefs, practices, and health literacy on the quality of patient care that is received. The challenge is figuring out which tools and frameworks will best deliver cultural competency training in our curricula.

In 2020, Brottman and colleagues evaluated the biomedical literature to determine how topics related to diversity and inclusion, including implicit bias, patient advocacy, and cultural care of diverse patient populations, were being integrated into the health professional curriculum. They specifically focused on what strategies were being used to improve the cultural competency-based knowledge, attitudes, values, and skills of students, and they found that the most widely used cultural competency model was the Campinha-Bacote's Process of Cultural Competence in the Delivery of Healthcare Services. Campinha-Bacote's model focuses on the development of cultural competency as a process within the five constructs of *cultural awareness, knowledge, skills, encounters,* and *desires.* Additionally, the Purnell Model for Cultural Competency, initially designed for nursing students, offers a framework to assess an individual's cultural experiences through the lens of family, community, and global society.

Although developed for medical students, the Tool for Assessing Cultural Competence Training (TACCT) can be used to assess the breadth and depth of cultural competency content within the curricula. The revised, validated 42-item tool evaluates programmatic course teaching within six domains: health disparities, community strategies, bias/stereotyping, communication skills specific to cross-cultural communication, use of interpreters, and self-reflection/culture of medicine.

When used to assess courses across a curriculum, TACCT provides a complete map of the academic program and identifies gaps in content areas or within specific domains. Overlaps and duplications in the curriculum can also be identified. The authors of TACCT suggest that the tool can also be utilized for faculty development, needs assessment, curriculum assessment, or curricular inventory. Data generated from using TACCT can inform your strategic planning process to ensure that the educational experience is robust and appropriately prepares the learner to achieve cultural competency programmatic goals. It should be noted that no tool is perfect and that TACCT does not determine the amount of time dedicated to the delivery of cultural competency content, nor does it assess the quality of the faculty creating the content.

Another common question that comes up in the age of curricular density and hoarding is, *How much cultural competency content is sufficient to prepare our students to be able to provide culturally sensitive care with a focus on promoting health equity?* The quick answer is this is a life-long journey that never ends. The longer answer is scaffolding and building in the curriculum until a point of saturation is necessary. This question has also been explored in the biomedical lecture, which has explored various durations of training in healthcare professions schools, ranging from single short-term interventions of less than an hour to full-day workshops, full-semester courses, and interventions spanning the entire curriculum.

What seems clear to me is that if we want to ensure that these concepts have been fully understood and can be utilized by our learners, we need a healthy amount of integration throughout the entirety of our curricula. For example, we can create a foundational course that provides language and knowledge at an introductory level in the first year of the program. Then, throughout the rest of the program, we can incorporate active learning assignments, group activities, and hands-on lab experiences to reinforce these concepts and help students master the skills. We should understand that changes in attitudes and beliefs, as well as effective communication skills, come with time, and so we should not expect a one-off course or elective to fully prepare our students to be culturally competent providers. Some suggestions of topics to cover didactically are:

- **Social determinants of health (SDOH):** Social, political, economic, and environmental factors that can influence the well-being and health outcomes of individuals and communities.

- **Health disparities:** Differences in rates of health outcomes, quality, and access based on factors such as race, ethnicity, gender, socioeconomic status, or geography.

- **Intersectionality:** How several aspects of a person's identity (e.g., gender, class, race, ethnicity, etc.) can interact to affect their healthcare outcomes and/or experiences.

- **Implicit bias:** Unconscious beliefs or attitudes held by healthcare professionals toward certain individuals or groups that can negatively impact their communication, decisions, or interactions with patients, leading to negative health experiences or outcomes.

- **Cross-cultural communication:** Understanding and navigating the cultural nuances, beliefs, values, and communication styles of individuals from diverse cultures using various models of communication.

- **Migrant and refugee health/global health:** Addressing the cultural and social aspects that affect health during migration or displacement.

- **Racial equity:** The chance for all individuals of any race to access high quality healthcare and optimal health.

- **Disability inclusion:** Ensuring individuals with disabilities are given appropriate accommodation and care that properly address their needs and differences.

- **Sexual and gender minority health:** Culturally affirming care for individuals from the LGBTQ+ community, including but not limited to transgender individuals.

As I worked to integrate topics into my curriculum and course delivery, I found that structuring activities is just as important as the topics addressed. Using a three-phase format with an introduction, activity, and debriefing segment allows for predictability and deepening of understanding. Despite popular belief, I have also found that the debriefing should take the longest time, not the actual activity. Think of debriefing as where the reflection and magical "aha" moments happen. Also, don't save debriefing for the very end of your teaching; sprinkle it throughout the planned activities, and this is not just for your clinical practice coursework! Continuous exposure reinforces knowledge and opportunities to engage. Allow your students to soak in and integrate the ideas, concepts, and feelings they experienced and received.

Another best practice I can share is to integrate these activities into your curriculum as both required and elective offerings. We should not just implement cultural competence topics randomly but rather map them to our curricular outcomes, scaffold them throughout the program, and, even better, spiral them from the first to the last year of training. We should also consider various types of assessment, which are also linked to learning objectives, to determine how students are filling in their learning gaps and mastering their understanding.

Ultimately, we want all of our students to walk across the graduation stage saying, *"I feel confident I can address SDOH, advocate for my patients, practice humility, and advance health equity."* Ask yourself, do you think your students would say this confidently on graduation day? Having an interdisciplinary approach reinforces that these topics are not limited to only one health profession or discipline to address. It is not just case managers, social workers, and physicians who should know how to address social determinants of health and health literacy or have effective cross-cultural communication skills with patients; rather, it demands a collective effort from all disciplines.

Case Study: A Foundational Course in Health Equity and Cultural Care

Using TACCT, I was eager to investigate gaps in my own curriculum. The goal was to create a foundational course to help students understand concepts related to these topics through attaining self-awareness, cultural sensitivity, cultural adaptability, and respect for others. Eventually, I developed a required course focused on key concepts of public health as they relate to the role of pharmacists in disease prevention, health promotion, and health equity. Students are introduced to concepts of health disparities, social determinants of health, health belief models, health literacy, and constructs of culturally competent care as they think about healthcare through a patient's eyes. Students are also expected to understand the necessary adaptations to healthcare delivery to promote equitable health for all. They were expected to acquire both generic and specific cultural knowledge that reflects an understanding of the diversity that exists between and within populations through lectures, group discussions, self-reflective activities, and exams.

My goal was to shift from a purely biomedical focus on illness to a more holistic integration of social justice, cultural competence, and human rights by examining the dynamics of power, oppression, and privilege in our healthcare system. This was the application of a more "people-centered" view of health. Several years into delivering this course, I have received overwhelmingly positive evaluations

"Cultural Competence" in the Curriculum

from students with comments like, *"Dr. Arif fostered a safe and inclusive environment, which allowed students to feel comfortable in class discussions about topics that are often avoided. Using real-life examples and case studies, she helped us grasp the roots of health disparities in America. Dr. Arif not only taught us about these issues but also inspired us to get involved and find solutions, emphasizing the importance of providing unbiased and discrimination-free care to every patient."*

I learned that there needs to be flexibility when adding these types of topics to the curriculum. Historically, these topics have been seen as more nuanced or complex than clinical courses, reinforcing the idea that cultural competency is secondary rather than essential to patient care. I also learned that there is often a feeling of limited "expertise" or capacity for faculty to take on teaching such topics. This is where I learned not to be afraid to reach out to other healthcare faculty in different disciplines to assist with my efforts to elevate this content. This also helped me alleviate the burnout I was feeling.For example, you could involve clinical psychology faculty to assist with content development and instruction around trauma-informed care. You could even consider recruiting community members who work within gender and sexual minority health to guest lecture on the provision of LGBTQ+ affirming healthcare in your course. Do not hesitate to explore unconventional avenues to support content development and delivery; after all, this content resonates universally across all healthcare disciplines.

Frameworks for Developing Culturally Competent Curricula

There has been a lot of criticism of existing cultural competence training programs for their simplistic approaches—boiling down cultural differences to mere lists of what to do and not to do with diverse patients. In medical education, Kripalani and colleagues have offered nine recommendations for curricular integration that have also been adapted across other health profession programs:

- Use frameworks like Fowkes and Berlin's LEARN (Listen, Explain, Acknowledge, Recommend, Negotiate) guidelines; Kleinman-Eisenberg-Good's questionnaire; and Kagawa-Singer and Kassim-Lakha's RISK (Resources, Identity, Skills, and Knowledge) framework to assess the student's cross-cultural skills.

- Use interactive educational methods (standardized patient encounters, role-play, and self-reflective journal assignments).

- Provide direct faculty observation and feedback by recording patient encounter sessions, reviewing the recordings with students, and providing feedback to students on their ability to elicit culturally appropriate information from patients.

- Discuss cultural competence throughout clinical education rather than in isolated workshops.

- Get buy-in from the top by seeking the support of medical school deans and course directors and forming a cultural competency team to help drive curricular integration.

- Promote cultural diversity among medical students and at all levels of the medical school.

- Involve an increasing number of "opinion leaders" as physician champions to disseminate culturally appropriate behaviors and approaches to patient care, minimize the racial discord between providers and patients, and increase the uptake of cultural competency education into the curriculum.

- Develop a cadre of dedicated faculty as preceptors to encourage routine inclusion of discussions on multicultural issues during patient care.
- Make it a "real science" by encouraging research on health disparities and evaluating cultural competence in medical education using Objective Structured Clinical Examinations (OSCE) and videotaped or audiotaped clinical encounters.

Another framework for cultural competency training is offered in graduate nursing education through Clark and colleagues' six core cultural competencies:

- Prioritize the social and cultural factors that affect health in designing and delivering care across multiple contexts.
- Construct socially and empirically derived cultural knowledge of people and populations to guide practice and research.
- Assume leadership in developing, implementing, and evaluating culturally competent nursing and other healthcare services.
- Transform healthcare systems to address social justice and health disparities.
- Provide leadership to educators and members of the healthcare or research team in learning, applying, and evaluating continuous cultural competence development.
- Conduct culturally competent scholarship that can be utilized in practice.

Using several of these frameworks myself, I developed my first intercultural-focused elective course nearly a decade ago. I called it *Health promotion and disease prevention across cultures,* and I went on to publish the results as a means to disseminate a methodology for training pharmacy students to provide culturally sensitive care through a tailored, whole-person-centered approach. We included weekly workshops alongside didactic lectures focused on addressing cardiovascular health disparities in Chicago communities. This included offering health access and awareness interventions for Black, Latine, Arab, and Asian communities.

Students were expected to not only practice their clinical skills related to hypertension, diabetes, and dyslipidemia management but also apply their growing cross-cultural communication skills. The active learning activities I used were based on shared resources I pooled alongside colleagues across several institutions who were also engaged in cultural competency training. Over the course of 10 weeks, we observed an overall increase in students' confidence in their abilities to provide culturally sensitive care and to communicate with a diverse patient population facing language barriers and low health literacy.

In the cultural competency space, there is no need to reinvent the wheel. Find collaborators and a "tribe" of others who will help support you and share resources mutually. Through shared expertise with colleagues across the country, I've discovered activities such as Global Beads, Trading Places, and BaFa BaFa (along with many others that I've included for you in the appendix of this book). In hindsight, I found this to be a major factor in my success as an educator, evolving in my own pedagogical approaches to teaching intercultural care.

Elevating Justice in Our Teaching

It is one thing to differentiate between equality and equity; it is another to describe to learners the need to strive for justice in healthcare. Justice in healthcare delivery means fair and equitable distribution of healthcare resources, opportunities, and outcomes, regardless of someone's socio-economic status, ethnicity, gender, or other factors. This concept can also be linked to *distributive justice*, where our goal is to minimize disparities and promote equal access to healthcare services.

Elevating the conversation around justice gives our students the opportunity to internalize the tenets of cultural humility and patient advocacy. It carves a path for them as rising healthcare professionals to understand the *who, what,* and *how* when addressing the causes of inequities in order to respond to present-day health injustice problems.

Brazilian educational theorist, Paulo Freire's *Pedagogy of the Oppressed* introduces the concept of "critical pedagogy," which is often described as "problem-posing education." In this approach, students delve into conditions of inequity and actively challenge the established norms through collaborative dialogue and a shared commitment to justice and liberation. For instance, instead of presenting learners with health disparities as mere facts, we raise their awareness of the patterns of inequity by encouraging them to critically question why systems uphold oppressive practices. This process is what Freire describes as building "critical consciousness." The literature acknowledges the significance of incorporating critical pedagogy and health justice studies into medical education. It enhances trainees' abilities to respond with compassion to structural biases within the health sector when they consider political, cultural, and social determinants of health.

Chapter 20

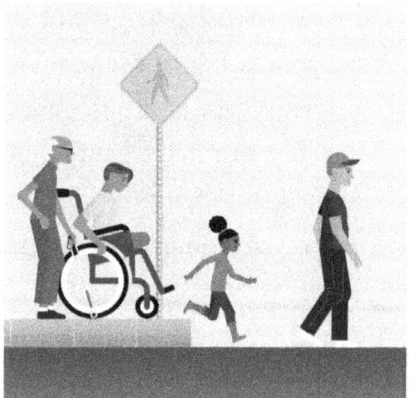
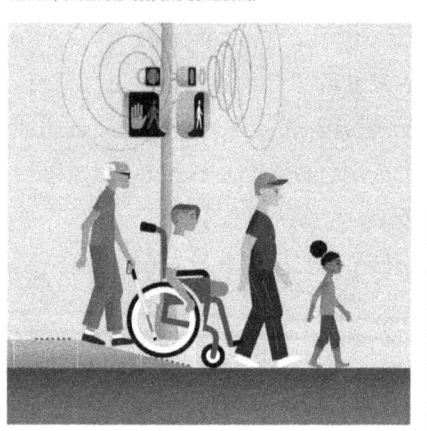

EQUALITY: Everyone gets the same – regardless if it's needed or right for them.

EQUITY: Everyone gets what they need – understanding the barriers, circumstances, and conditions.

FIGURE 8: EQUALITY AND EQUITY

I find this image (Figure 8) to be a powerful tool to practice critical pedagogy and encourage my students to engage in discussions about inequities within our contemporary healthcare system at the intersections of justice. I ask them, *"What are the problems with equality-only based approaches in healthcare? Who do you think constructed the curb and light fixtures? What assumptions are ingrained in our actions when we work with communities facing oppression, disadvantage, displacement, or language barriers? How can we leverage our own social authority and power to address upstream environmental and social conditions that impact a patient's health status?"* Exploring these questions not only stimulates critical thinking and dialogue on the distinctions between equity and equality but also underscores our collective and individual social responsibility to address health access and system inequities. Until we dismantle common causes of injustices—like racism, classism, and sexism—our pedagogy necessitates a justice-oriented approach.

Key Takeaways:

1. Center cultural humility over competency in your teaching to promote the learner's ongoing self-awareness and learning.

2. Shift from patient-centered to "people-" or "person-centered" care to consider the structural competency needed to have a holistic approach when addressing social, economic, and political influences on healthcare.

3. Strategic planning when integrating inclusive content into curricula can include using models for cultural competence that emphasize ongoing, scaffolded education and interdisciplinary collaboration for culturally competent healthcare professionals.

4. Resources to assist you with implementing this chapter using pedagogical tools can be found via the QR code in the appendix.

CHAPTER 21

•

Health Equity in Experiential Teaching

*"Health cannot be a question of income;
it is a fundamental human right."*
—Nelson Mandela

The Latin word "docco" is where the word "doctor" is derived from, and it means "to teach." We often see in allopathic medicine that the act of teaching our patients is not prioritized in a clinician's busy day-to-day activities. Educating our patients and enhancing their self-efficacy is crucial to practicing as culturally sensitive providers. Ultimately, we want our learners to help educate their patients and communities and meet them where they are. This means, as mindful preceptors, we must guide our learners to be responsive to patient needs over their self-interest and center health equity in our experiential teaching. We must model these principles through our daily actions.

Hands-on experiences, such as practical clinical rotations, offer students more than just cultural insights. It gives them opportunities to apply classroom learning directly to patient care as they collaborate with under-resourced communities facing significant health disparities. The good news is that the current

Chapter 21

generation of trainees are excited and motivated to address health injustices but don't necessarily have the words or tools to mobilize into action. *Our goal is to build their capacity to turn their passion into meaningful, equitable change.*

By advocating for health equity in your precepting, you directly shape a healthcare workforce that embraces social justice and is better prepared to serve diverse communities. Although healthcare is deeply affected by discrimination, the way we frame the issue is crucial when addressing inequalities with our learners. By adopting a comprehensive perspective and valuing diverse disciplines and community viewpoints, we can diminish inequities through analytical methods and innovative strategies.

I strongly advocate for not only recognizing disparities but also using multidisciplinary, team-driven approaches to drive transformative, systemic improvements. All hands on deck, literally, with this one. No one specialty holds a spot in the driver's seat.

We have established that health disparities are not random occurrences. They are rooted in systemic inequities related to race, ethnicity, socioeconomic status, gender, sexual orientation, disability, and other marginalized identities. Think of integrating health equity concepts into your precepting as advocacy work. For example, acknowledge the current controversies in race-based clinical algorithms or results of clinical trials and discuss what activism would look like to address these domains. When working with patients with limited English proficiency, encourage your trainees to use interpretive services to identify challenges in access. When we aim for our trainees to better understand these systemic issues and work toward addressing them, we collectively contribute to dismantling systems of oppression and advocating for equitable policies and practices within healthcare and society at large.

In the book *The Death Gap*, health equity advocate and author Dr. David Ansell explores the issue of health disparities between different socioeconomic groups in the United States. He argues in his book that there is a significant gap in health outcomes between those who are affluent and those who are economically disadvantaged. He discusses the root reasons for this gap, including race, income, and education level. He also highlights the impact of systemic racism, inadequate access to healthcare, and food insecurity on health disparities. For example, he illustrates a 13-year mortality gap between residents in the Loop of Chicago and those in West Garfield Park, just 5 miles away. *This shows our zip codes, not genetic codes, make a greater difference in our survival.* The book emphasizes the need for policy codes to address social drivers of health. Solutions, such as expanding access to healthcare and improving the quality of education and housing, are also suggested.

When I first read Ansell's book I saw a compelling analysis of the complex and interrelated factors that contribute to health disparities in the United States and a roadmap for addressing these critical issues. It also provides a foundation for where health professional students can start addressing health inequities in the communities they serve, including some of the following:

- **Education and awareness:** Educate themselves and others about the social determinants of health and how they impact health disparities. This knowledge can help them identify and address health inequities.

- **Advocacy:** Advocate for policies that promote health equity at the local, state, and national levels. They can participate in advocacy campaigns and work with policymakers to promote policies that address health inequities.

- **Culturally competent care:** Integrate frameworks such as the Minority Stress Model, the Lens of Systemic Oppression, and the Health Belief Model to provide care that is sensitive to the cultural and social needs of their patients.

- **Research:** Explore how they can engage in health disparity-based research by working with researchers at various clinical sites to identify the underlying causes of health inequities. They can also use their research to advocate for policies that address health disparities. Medical students who did corridor work in West Garfield Park in Chicago found a 25% decline in population from 2000 to 2010, with only 57% of residents having primary care doctors vs. 73% living in the Loop.

- **Community engagement:** Engage with community organizations in their local neighborhoods that work on health equity issues. They can volunteer their time and expertise to help these organizations with their programs and initiatives.

Case Study: Social Responsibility of Community Assessment and Engagements

> *"I will not walk away from the people and communities whom I love deeply."*
> —Linda Sarsour

A few years into working as a pharmacist at Rush University Medical Center, I learned about their involvement in the Westside United Initiative. It was an effort that began in 2017 to improve access to mental health services and promote community wellness programs. It is a tale of the intentionality of healthcare systems like

Rush, working with the 10 communities around them. The story showed us how to avoid falling into the trap of over-promising and under-delivering when deploying resources and support to communities of color. The initiative is an important step toward addressing health disparities and promoting health equity in Chicago's West Side, in collaboration with six other hospitals and health systems. By focusing on bridging the gap in health disparities, the initiative aims to address social determinants of health that affect the West Side community. The goal is to improve health outcomes and economic opportunities for residents, with efforts concentrated on five key areas:

- **Economic vitality:** The initiative aims to promote economic development and create job opportunities for West Side residents.

- **Neighborhood and physical environment:** The initiative seeks to improve the safety and walkability of the community, increase access to healthy food, and support affordable housing.

- **Education:** The initiative aims to improve educational outcomes for West Side youth and promote lifelong learning opportunities for adults.

- **Healthcare:** The initiative seeks to increase access to healthcare services and improve the quality of care provided to West Side residents.

- **Collaboration:** The initiative promotes collaboration among community organizations, healthcare providers, and other stakeholders to address health disparities in the West Side community.

Sharing this initiative with my learners on rotation allowed them to strategize in integrating these focus areas when designing their care plans and engaging with the community directly. This allowed for richer discussions and contextualization of knowledge about social determinants of health. It also gave the chance for my clerkship learners to craft solutions as culturally sensitive and patient-centered providers on a mission to reduce health disparities and contribute to healthier communities.

Social Determinants of Health & Community Engagement

We should explore student interests and get them out of their own bubble about discussing what is involved in the process of achieving equitable health outcomes for medically underserved populations. The U.S. Department of Health and Human Services defines medically underserved populations as communities that include: 1) racial and ethnic minorities; 2) people with physical disabilities; 3) individuals with low income; or 4) those living in rural areas according to census data.

During my rotation, I have learners explore using online maps (see Appendix) to determine social vulnerability, social determinants of health, and other health access points in not just the community we serve at my hospital but within their own home communities or cities. Highlighting these points helps students, for example, see the impact of historical factors like redlining on the care provided to patients and populations. I also expect my students to address the patient's social determinants of health within their patient presentations and in any formal case presentations. Highlighting the barriers to access, cost, or community support often falls on our social workers but is essential to any treatment plan. This also becomes a launching point to discuss what the responsibility of each healthcare provider is to create initiatives and engage with communities to advance equitable care.

Providing learners with reflection points to bring them more self-awareness, as well as networking and research opportunities, is key. The introspection starts with learners reflecting on questions around topics like:

- **Community investments and pathways:** How do they themselves define "community?" How would they approach a community needs assessment (e.g., schools, hospitals, clinics, pharmacies, grocery stores, etc.)? What tools do we, as educators, need to provide and guide them through to complete such assessments? How do our learners engage with communities, get buy-in, and build sustainable collaboration?

- **Organizational approaches:** What (if any) programs are available at your site/institution to assist populations which have been identified to be more vulnerable to poor health outcomes and/or lost to follow-up care? How are patients enrolled in these programs, and how does the program address disparities in care? Is there community engagement in these plans? How are barriers in digital health and issues of technology literacy addressed?

- **Patient-related:** What is their access to high quality healthcare? Are there any charity care initiatives offered? What is the use of certified interpreters?

- **Workforce-related:** What anti-racism and inclusive behavior training is offered to the healthcare workforce? What cultural responsiveness training is offered? This is where you can share with your learners if you've ever witnessed patients being treated differently or disrespectfully by providers due to their social identities.

- **Advocacy:** What is their role as a dentist, a pharmacist, a physician, or any other healthcare professional to be a facilitator of change and leader in healthcare equity initiatives?

Don't feel you need to tackle everything at once. Begin by recognizing that your commitment to health equity is not just a responsibility; it's a powerful opportunity to transform the future of healthcare. After reading this chapter, reflect on the opportunities within your current practice that you can leverage to actively engage your learners as advocates for healthier communities.

Key Takeaways:

1. Hands-on experiences offer learners the opportunity to apply classroom knowledge to direct patient care in underserved communities facing significant health disparities.

2. When we advocate for health equity as preceptors, we shape a healthcare workforce that embraces social justice and is better prepared to serve diverse communities.

3. Integration of health equity concepts into precepting is a form of advocacy that encourages trainees to understand systemic issues contributing to health disparities and work toward addressing them through community engagement and social responsibility.

4. Resources to assist you with implementing this chapter using pedagogical tools can be found via the QR code in the appendix.

CHAPTER 22

•

Case-Based Learning and Simulations

"We may have different religions, different languages, different colored skin, but we all belong to one human race."
—Kofi Annan

    We know that classroom engagement is key to being a good teacher, but I want to make a case for how engagement helps us cultivate belonging and can shift us into being more inclusive and equitable. When examining the most effective methods for developing a student's cultural competence and humility within a school of health professions, it becomes clear that the traditional lecture format falls short. Active learning strategies have been found to be more effective than traditional lectures in promoting cultural competency. Numerous educational studies have reinforced strategies like discussion groups, reflections, case-based learning, simulations, cultural immersion, videos, readings, and, to a lesser extent, written papers and presentations to better enhance learning outcomes. Active learning allows learners to engage with our content at their personal level of insight, rather than just passively talking about it.

Chapter 22

Hafferty's taxonomy of curricula, described as formal, informal, and hidden curriculum, has been used to describe the integration of cultural competence as it relates to clinical preceptor training and professional development tools needed for faculty. The formal cultural competence curriculum allows students to understand historical and social interplay, develop communication skills during clinical interactions, and improve self-awareness. The informal curriculum is an approach that integrates cultural competence during interpersonal interactions that are not necessarily related to classroom-based lectures; but are rather observed among student peers and faculty outside the classroom. The *hidden curriculum* consists of the unspoken rules, values, and norms taught through institutional culture.

Approaches to Diversifying Case-Based Learning

Historically, health science education has relied on case-based learning (CBL). Most healthcare educators concur that CBL effectively builds practical skills and knowledge. But I am often asked, *"What is the best way to infuse cultural competency into CBL?"* I suggest starting by reflecting on the most memorable clinical scenarios you've encountered in your past real-life patient experiences. Reflect on which patients made you pause and think about unique cultural, social, environmental, or demographic characteristics. Integrating diversity in patient cases mirrors the reality of our healthcare landscape. Rather than shielding our trainees from these factors, it prepares them for the complexities they will encounter in their practice, including issues related to provider bias, social determinants of health, and health literacy.

I have also been asked if we should diversify identities in all our patient cases. Instructors often ask this because they want to

Case-Based Learning and Simulations

honor the varying diversity and lived experiences seen in real-life patient care, but they are afraid to perpetuate biases or stereotypes. This worry drives some educators to remove all forms of identity from their cases in an effort to be more "inclusive." In my view, this approach might inadvertently have the opposite effect by reinforcing dominant narrative experiences, as discussed in Chapter 5. Stripping away all identities could unintentionally reinforce the *hidden curriculum*—the incidental learning occurring within our programs, influenced by the content we choose to include or exclude. These learning experiences are often based on assumptions and the instructors' own lived experiences, rooted in social cognitive theory. This hidden curriculum may impact the development of students' knowledge, skills, attitudes, and behaviors, either positively or negatively, influencing their learning journey.

So, how does this all relate to diversifying our patient cases? Well, we, as humans, make a lot of assumptions, and when diverse representation is absent, this may undermine our efforts for inclusion and affirmation. If cases are largely undefined, it is seen that healthcare students tend to automatically visualize patients based on their personal experiences, backgrounds, or dominant societal norms and narratives. So basically, we could unintentionally teach from a White, cisgendered, heteronormative, ableist lens case. On the other end, we also make assumptions and can perpetuate negative stereotypes when diverse representation is showcased without any historical context (for example, a BIPOC patient is presented as a single parent or uninsured). What we should consider is that adding diversifying factors to our cases without careful consideration may tokenize or reinforce population-level stereotypes.

So yes, diversifying cases can be valuable, but we also have to create space for discussing relevance and social/historical context alongside CBL. For instance, you can consider embedding discussions about social determinants of health into your patient cases. Explore how factors such as education, transportation, food, housing, and safety impact health outcomes. This encourages students to consider the broader context of patient care.

Moreover, presenting the epidemiology of a disease accurately is essential for comprehending and addressing public health concerns. However, it should be presented without perpetuating stereotypes or reinforcing biases. For instance, while sickle cell disease is more prevalent among Black patients in the United States, it's essential to question whether every case needs to be framed around a Black patient. Similarly, must a patient with HIV always be associated with the gay male community? The key is, when discussing a patient's case, we ensure that information is presented in a fair, unbiased, and scientifically valid manner.

RB is a 65 year old male who presents with cough and fatigue... sound familiar? Get creative and expand beyond conventional categories like race, gender, or age when diversifying patient cases. A moment of insight struck me during a healthcare conference where a transgender patient shared an unsettling experience at a physician's office. Despite seeking treatment for a broken foot, the physician excessively focused on the patient's medical transition. This prompted me to consider a more creative approach to case design, intentionally including identifiers like transgender, disabled, or obese that are wholly irrelevant to the patient's complaints or diagnosis. The aim is to underscore how, even when unrelated to the patient's actual care needs, we often tend to hyper-focus on such aspects and make assumptions. This strategy can serve as a powerful tool to raise awareness about unconscious biases and encourage a more holistic and person-centered approach.

Engaging and obtaining perspectives from diverse populations with lived experiences, including members of our campus community and can serve to enrich CBL. Involving faculty and students from underrepresented backgrounds in the case development process allows for valuable insights into the nuances of diverse patient experiences and helps create more authentic and culturally sensitive cases. Diverse perspectives contributing to case creation open the door for dynamic curricular plans and the potential for co-creation with students. Additionally, I regularly hold intentional time for questions that arise from deploying my patient cases in assessments. This provides me with a valuable opportunity to gather feedback from students about how the questions were received and what further refinements are needed for my assessment questions.

Approaches to Diversifying Patient Simulations

"I believed this simulation mirrored real-life situations. My patient was going through an emotional time. Typically, in clinical simulations, patients are there solely for drug or diagnostic information. This patient simulated encounter represented the emotional aspect of healthcare, illustrating how we, as healthcare providers, need to be there for our patients."

"This experience offered a valuable opportunity to gain firsthand experience in handling diverse encounters before entering the real-world healthcare setting. It allowed me to develop a deeper understanding of the importance of flexibility and adaptability when caring for patients with varying needs, ultimately preparing me for the challenges I may face in my future medical career."

My students shared these reflections immediately after completing a standardized patient encounter in our clinical skills lab. The acting patient in this encounter was emotional due to a recent breast cancer diagnosis and was reluctant to inform their family or take prescription medications for prevention of chemo-induced emesis due to spiritual beliefs. Students were instructed to elicit pertinent cultural information and counsel the patient, addressing their medication-related questions using cross-cultural communication skills, which required a deep understanding of the patient's health beliefs and concerns. The rubric was shared ahead of the simulated patient encounter and closely aligned with these expectations. They were tasked with applying frameworks such as SOLER, a non-verbal counseling approach, and LEARN, a verbal framework, to overcome cultural communication barriers. The simulation also allowed students to apply the Health Belief Model by tailoring their communication strategies to align with the patient's beliefs and attitudes. The objective was to assess the patient's health literacy and provide effective care. While I had several deliverables for the students, this simulation, offered before their final year of clinical rotations, provided a valuable opportunity for them to demonstrate their ability to apply multiple frameworks and models in a simulated safe environment.

Simulation-based pedagogy has been used across many disciplines to promote self-awareness, critical thinking, and problem-solving using trained actors in what mimics a real-world setting. More broadly, simulation exercises can also include role-playing with standardized patients, the use of OSCEs, discussion groups, or even mixed models of these strategies. Discussion groups, consisting of 8-10 students, and panel discussions in larger groups have also been reported as effective learning opportunities for students to practice skill building. In more recent years, leveraging digital platforms to simulate telehealth encounters have also been utilized to reflect the evolving landscape of virtual healthcare delivery.

Case-Based Learning and Simulations

Many clinician training programs use trained standardized patients to portray patient scenarios for the instruction and assessment of clinical skills in medical students, residents, and other allied health professionals. However, programs striving to integrate more diversity into their patients' cases may face challenges in recruiting enough standardized patients with specific identities due to geographic location or other ethical barriers. The question arises: *Is it appropriate to have actors who may not have a particular identity play a scripted role for the sake of student learning? For example, should an actor who identifies as being straight portray a patient who is gay or transgender? Or can a standardized patient portray a patient with a spinal cord injury in a wheelchair?* When hiring actors, if the representation of a specific identity is not available, you can consider enhancing other aspects of diversity—for instance, religious beliefs, health literacy, socioeconomic background, relationship status, or veteran status. It is crucial to assess whether actors are over-representing or stereotyping that identity and address these issues appropriately. Involving individuals with the relevant identity in the creation of scenarios helps ensure that portrayals are both respectful and accurate. Seeking feedback from learners about how cases landed for them can provide valuable insights and pathways for improvement.

Reflective exercises following OSCEs are essential, prompting students to consider how their responses or interactions would have been different if the patient had a different identity. Or you could ask students to complete a post-simulation reflection to express what role they see healthcare professionals playing in promoting health equity as it relates to the patient encounter they experienced. I have also held large group debriefs to discuss how insights gained regarding cultural sensitivity can be applied to improve care for future patients from diverse backgrounds.

Chapter 22

I encourage you to reflect on what you have learned about your own cases or approaches to writing cases as you have read this text. Get creative with your existing simulations to integrate a patient advocacy component that challenges students to navigate situations where patients face discrimination, stigma, or barriers to care. Have them practice being an upstander during an interdisciplinary team meeting or even have them practice how they would react to a biased patient (see Chapter 19).

Bringing Lived Experiences to Life

I was once discussing Toya Wolfe's book, *Last Summer on State Street* with a nursing educator colleague. She described the profound insights offered in the book as Wolfe grew up in the 1990s in one of Chicago's most perilous housing projects. In the book, Wolfe shared her experience: *"Maybe the worst part about growing up in public housing is that people think your body is public too. That even before you are born, your Black body already belongs to the owners of the land."* While not all our learners could know what this felt like, presenting these lived experiences to them provides the opportunity to explore the depths of real-life narratives vividly within our classrooms. We can do this with so many other books, podcasts, or even by inviting actual patients into our classes to share their journeys and challenges in the healthcare system. Encouraging students to reflect on such poignant quotes or stories gives them a tangible connection to other people's realities—an education that transcends the pages of a book or a second-hand recount. Consider using multimedia elements like videos, audio recordings, or patient testimonials to provide a more comprehensive understanding of cultural nuances and diverse healthcare experiences.

Key Takeaways:

1. Active learning methods, like discussions and simulations, over traditional lectures to enhance cultural competence in health professional education, emphasizing engagement and practical skill development.

2. Diversifying case-based learning should reflect healthcare realities, avoid perpetuating biases, and consider the impact of the hidden curriculum.

3. Incorporating lived experiences through multimedia, patient stories, and reflections is essential to provide a comprehensive understanding of cultural nuances and diverse healthcare experiences, contributing to a more inclusive educational environment.

4. Resources to assist you with implementing this chapter using pedagogical tools can be found via the QR code in the appendix.

CHAPTER 23

•

Decolonizing the Curriculum

"You can't be the doctor if you are the disease."
—Mi'kmaw Elder Kji Keptin Alex Denny

Contemporary times have a spotlight on diversifying everything from our recruitment efforts to content in our health profession programs. What is really needed beyond the diversification of our curricula and training programs is to elevate our goal and shift to *decolonizing* our curricula. The systems we currently operate within have been designed to marginalize or unfairly under-resource people not because of their height, favorite color, or model of the car they drive but rather due to factors like belonging to racial or ethnic minority groups, having a disability, their country of origin, or their socioeconomic class. Decolonization is a proactive, ongoing process that acknowledges historical systems of oppression and seeks to humanize those who have been marginalized.

The idea of "decolonization' first appeared in academic discourse in 2011 and was rooted in creating more inclusive humanities curricula based on the "Why Is My Curriculum So White?" protests organized by university students in the 1990s. If we apply the "SHIFT" principles to our contemporary curricula, it provokes us to move beyond just inclusive teaching to examining how we present race and other marginalized identities in our classroom discussions and materials. We need to go beyond merely updating dermatological images in our medical education materials to include diverse skin tones. We must also address our academic culture that excludes Black, Indigenous, and other historically marginalized groups from our mainstream teaching. What we focus on in our curricula sends a message to students about who matters and who doesn't. But the elephant in the room is that racial anxiety is real. In the process of addressing racism, White individuals often worry they will be perceived as racist, and BIPOC individuals are worried they will encounter racism. Grappling with both responses is challenging, but conflating these emotional struggles as equal is a product of white supremacy.

If the mention of white supremacy evoked any sort of discomfort, take a deep breath. It is crucial to grasp that white supremacy as an ideology is not confined to individuals of just White descent but is a set of beliefs based on the unfounded notion that there is a superiority of lighter-skinned, or "white" human races over other racial groups. It is possible for people, including those from BIPOC backgrounds, to inadvertently perpetuate certain aspects of white supremacy due to internalized biases or societal conditioning. If we want to decolonize our curriculum, we must first acknowledge this complex interplay of emotions and societal ideologies in order to shift a more nuanced understanding of the impact of systemic racism in healthcare education.

If you identify as being White, take some time to reflect on the following: *How do I feel about my responsibility to challenge White-centered norms in my professional life? What discomfort do I feel when I reflect on my relationship with Whiteness, and how can I use that discomfort as an opportunity for growth and learning?*

Anti-racist Pedagogy

"We must always attempt to lift as we climb."
—Angela Davis

The ultimate goal of decolonizing the curriculum is to create more inclusive and equitable educational spaces that promote critical thinking, empathy, and social justice, specifically through *anti-racist pedagogy*. This can involve incorporating perspectives and knowledge from diverse sources, engaging with Indigenous knowledge and epistemologies, and challenging dominant narratives that reinforce oppression and privilege in our healthcare settings. If we want to promote whole-person care, we must prioritize the needs and preferences of marginalized communities in medical care and work collaboratively with patients to co-create treatment plans that are responsive to their cultural backgrounds, values, and beliefs.

Decolonizing the curriculum is a process of re-evaluating and transforming our content and structures to challenge dominant perspectives, biases, and power dynamics that have historically always been present. This process involves critically examining the ways in which knowledge is created, taught, and validated within our institutions. Acknowledging and addressing the impact of colonization and systemic inequities on oppressed individuals and communities helps us incorporate diverse voices, perspectives, and histories that have been previously erased. Furthermore, decolonization of healthcare education requires an anti-racist approach by first acknowledging that racism exists and is rooted in choices that take place in everyday life, including educational environments and materials.

Chapter 23

A "colonized" health sciences curriculum refers to a program that has been influenced or shaped by colonial ideologies, biases, and perspectives, often resulting in the marginalization or exclusion of non-Western medical knowledge, practices, and cultural contexts. Here are some examples of features that may be found in a colonized health professions curriculum:

- **Eurocentric medical history:** The curriculum may primarily focus on the history of Western medicine, downplaying the contributions of non-Western medical systems and traditional healing practices.

- **Limited cultural competence training:** There may be insufficient emphasis on training students to understand and respect diverse cultural beliefs and health practices, leading to potential misunderstandings and misdiagnoses in cross-cultural healthcare interactions.

- **Biased research and evidence:** The curriculum may prioritize research from Western institutions, leading to a lack of evidence-based studies on health issues prevalent in non-Western populations. Emphasizing clinical trials that exclude racial and ethnic minorities, sexual and gender minorities, and those from socioeconomically disadvantaged backgrounds.

- **Neglecting Indigenous healing practices:** Traditional healing practices of Indigenous communities may be overlooked or dismissed as "folk medicine," devaluing their effectiveness and cultural significance.

- **Lack of diversity in faculty:** A colonized curriculum may have a predominantly White, Eurocentric faculty, resulting in a limited range of perspectives and expertise.

- **Underrepresentation of global health issues:** The curriculum may not adequately address the health challenges faced by under-resourced communities in developing countries or regions affected by historical colonialism.

- **Disregard for holistic medicine:** Non-Western approaches to health, which often emphasize holistic well-being, may be marginalized in favor of a more reductionist biomedical approach.

- **Overemphasis on Western pharmacology:** The curriculum may excessively focus on Western pharmaceuticals while neglecting the study of traditional remedies and herbal medicines used by different cultures.

- **Reinforcing health disparities:** A colonized curriculum might perpetuate health disparities by neglecting to address the social and systemic determinants of health that disproportionately impact communities of color and those experiencing disadvantage.

The Role that Race Plays in Healthcare

At a recent health equity conference I attended, a participant shared that they believed most healthcare professionals do not even know how to conceptualize, let alone contextualize, race and racism in medicine. They relayed that when they routinely ask their students and residents to define race, they are met with blank or uncomfortable stares. Why do so many not understand that race is a sociopolitical construct that is used to consolidate power in one group (e.g., social hierarchies) and disenfranchise others (e.g., limit access to resources or opportunities)? Why do countless numbers of healthcare professionals who have been practicing for decades still believe that race has a biological basis? I reflected on these questions and felt a relief as I read one of my student's entries after a lecture where we discussed how racism, not race, is the key driver of many health disparities. The second year medical student's entry provided a critical reevaluation of the role of race in healthcare we should all take note of:

Today's discussion prompted me to critically revisit the involvement I previously thought race had in healthcare. Previously, I thought that race was a conclusive demographic that could be used to think of pertinent diagnoses or conditions that are more prevalent in certain groups. However, after today's discussion, I am not sure that my previous views are completely accurate. Our discussion allowed me to begin to understand the amount of genetic diversity that exists within one race—so much so that saying a certain race is at higher risk for health problems still leaves us with a very broad group. This prompts me to wonder if there exists a point in including the patient's race to begin with. An example of this is the discussion we had on sickle cell anemia (SCA). While it may be argued that knowing your patient's race can help you determine whether or not your patient is at high risk of SCA, we would never base a diagnosis simply off of this. We would always look for a quantitative test to use, such as a peripheral blood smear. Since this is the case, I am left wondering why ever since high school biology it has been ingrained in my brain to associate high rates of SCA with African-American populations. How does this association actually help us in clinical practice?"

Race is a concept, not a fact...

We do not have a good handle on what race is in our society, so we shouldn't be surprised when our students are also left at a loss about the concept. We rarely discuss it openly and often make a deliberate effort to avoid the topic. But race undeniably influences numerous aspects of our lives. Determining someone's race often relies on observable phenotypic traits associated with particular ancestries, such as skin tone, speech patterns, facial features, or hair texture. We seldom question why we feel compelled to categorize people based on their physical traits, and this tendency has become deeply ingrained in our subconscious. Most of us know that this process is imperfect, and we often make mistakes. Race is a concept that our society revolves around, making it easy to make assumptions based on it. Even with my background in studying racial health inequities, I still find myself grappling with the concept.

First and foremost, it is important to recognize that race is a social construct that changes over time and varies in different geographical contexts. For example, as an Iraqi-American, I'm classified as "White" on the 2020 U.S. Census, even though my identity may not align with this label. In the past, race was influenced by factors such as social class and beliefs. It is evident that the notions of race and freedom were intertwined, contradicting the idea that "all men were created equal," as stated in the United States Constitution. The scientifically erroneous and morally reprehensible theory of eugenics, which advocated for "racial improvement" and controlled breeding, gained popularity in the early 20th century. Eugenicists across the globe believed they could enhance humanity and eliminate societal problems through genetic and hereditary means.

How do we integrate biological, environmental, and social factors that contribute to health disparities across racial and ethnic lines? It's important not to conflate ancestry with race. For instance, Ethiopian women are more likely to have sickle cell anemia than Black women in Georgia, despite both groups being of African descent. Epigenetics further complicates our understanding of these differences, making it clear that there is no simple, binary answer to addressing these disparities.

Chapter 23

Claiming to be "color-blind" (let's not get into how ableist this language is) in an attempt to address issues like racism only serves to erase the history of oppression and the underlying factors that have contributed to racial inequalities. Many White individuals might also see themselves as "raceless" due to their dominant social status. When we consider racial categorizations such as Black or White, it is important to acknowledge that these perspectives are primarily shaped by a complex history of colonization and slavery through a Euro-American lens and may not apply universally. Moreover, race is often confused with ethnicity, which is based on shared history, culture, and kinship and does not involve hierarchical distinctions. Ethnicity is grounded in our understanding of history and can exist within racial groups. For instance, in the United States, Asians are often grouped together racially despite comprising various distinct ethnic groups ranging from Chinese to Indo-Pakistani. Furthermore, Latino/a/x is not a race but an ethnic identity, as individuals from Latin America can belong to many different racial groups.

A conversation about decolonizing the curriculum is not complete without understanding the place that structural racism has played in higher education. Dr. David Williams from Harvard University describes structural racism as: *"an organized social system, in which the dominant racial group, based on an ideology of inferiority, categorizes and ranks people into social groups called 'races,' and uses its power to devalue, disempower, and differentially allocate valued societal resources and opportunities to groups defined as inferior."* These systems are shaped by political movements, our life-courses, and intersectional social identities, and they continue to evolve over time. The processes are mutually reinforcing and interdependent, and we see this reflected in our healthcare system. Being an anti-racist becomes so important because it goes beyond just being "not-racist." Psychologist and author Beverly Tatum put it so well when she couched the concept this way: *"I sometimes visualize the ongoing cycle of racism as a moving walkway at the airport. Active racist behavior is equivalent to walking fast on the conveyor belt ... Passive racist behavior is equivalent to standing still on the walkway. No overt effort is being made, but the conveyor belt moves the bystanders along to the same destination as those who are actively walking. Some of the bystanders may feel the motion of the conveyor belt, see the active racists ahead of them, and choose to turn around ... But unless they are walking actively in the opposite direction at a speed faster than the conveyor belt—unless they are actively anti-racist—they will find themselves carried along with the others."*

If we really want to decolonize our curricula, we must shift into operating from an anti-racist lens. Yes, this means you might feel some hesitation as you turn around on the conveyor belt; you might even risk tripping or losing your footing. But you take that risk for the sake of liberation. Acting as an ally means we recognize that liberation involves more than just resisting inequity—it requires actively working to dismantle all sources of injustice. Just as Beverly Tatum's analogy emphasizes the need for active effort to counteract racism, true liberation demands that we engage in deliberate and proactive steps to challenge and change the inequities that persist in our healthcare systems.

Case Study: Race-based Algorithms and Clinical Tools

The racialization of clinical calculators and decision-making tools should also be discussed with our learners in the clinical setting. Let's take the example of the MDRD equation, which is used to estimate the glomerular filtration rate in patients with chronic kidney disease. Recently, this test has been under scrutiny because it has not only been shown to overestimate kidney function for Black patients but also to have dire consequences like late diagnosis of chronic kidney disease and delayed transplant referrals. But how did we get to standardize the use of MDRD for kidney function in the first place? Blackness was assigned for the MDRD equation in a small sample size study based on the racist beliefs of White physicians centuries ago to uphold slavery of Black people and supported by only three small studies stating "on average, Black persons have greater muscle mass than White persons." Furthermore, the study assigned racial categorization to the subjects without explicit criteria.

MDRD isn't the only racialized tool that has caused harm. The article *Hidden in Plain Sight—Reconsidering the Use of Race Correction in Clinical Algorithms* highlights 13 race-based algorithms or clinical tools. While changing our habits can be challenging—especially later in our careers—we need to reassess all race-based decision tools, especially those developed with insufficient representation of racial minorities in their clinical datasets.

The lack of consistency in how we collect data is also complicating an already complicated system. We need a national stand for collecting self-identified REAL-D (race, ethnicity, language, and disability) data so we don't keep collecting inconsistent or missing data. This is both an operational and patient safety issue. We need to train our clinical staff and learners on how to collect this and start normalizing patient self-identification in both patient care and clinical trial settings. We must have active individuals and structural interventions to resolve these issues infused with empathy. While we speak about racism here, many of these discussions can also be applied to power dynamics found with sexual and gender minorities, religious minorities, migrants, and disability-based identities as well.

So, how do we go about decolonizing our curricula? The specific strategies and approaches will depend on the context and goals of our particular institutions and the communities we serve. Some strategies to start the process of decolonizing are:

- **Incorporating diverse perspectives and voices:** This could involve including readings and materials from a range of authors and scholars who represent diverse backgrounds and perspectives, including those from historically marginalized groups.

- **Engaging with Indigenous knowledge and epistemologies:** This could involve incorporating traditional knowledge systems, languages, and teachings from Indigenous cultures, as well as working collaboratively with Indigenous communities to co-create curriculum.

- **Critically examining dominant narratives:** This could involve challenging the ways in which certain histories, cultures, and worldviews have been privileged over others and exploring the ways in which these dominant narratives have been used to reinforce systems of oppression.

- **Centering marginalized voices and experiences:** This could involve prioritizing the experiences and perspectives of historically marginalized groups, such as people of color, sexual and gender minorities, and people with disabilities, and creating opportunities for these individuals to share their knowledge and expertise.

- **Fostering critical thinking and social justice:** This could involve incorporating activities and assignments that encourage students to critically examine power dynamics and inequalities that exist in medical care and to take action to address social and environmental justice issues that intersect with health. For example, in a role-play exercise centered on the toxic lead levels found in Flint, Michigan's water supply, students can adopt personas of key stakeholders—such as Flint residents, public health officials, or policymakers. They can explore the long-term health effects on the city's lower-income residents and explore the most effective response to environmental health threats.

- **Applying principles of anti-racist pedagogy:**
While inclusive pedagogy and anti-racist pedagogy both strive to promote critical thinking, empathy, and social responsibility among learners, anti-racist pedagogy challenges racist narratives, biases, and curriculum omissions. This could involve critical discussions of race in class, using diverse materials and resources, and addressing historical injustices. Ultimately, the goal is to empower students to be agents of change and contribute to a more just and equitable society through critical analysis of power dynamics, colonial histories, and institutional biases that perpetuate racial inequities in our healthcare system.

Decolonizing your curriculum should be considered an ever-evolving process that requires continuous reflection and adaptation. There is no one-and-done to this. While inclusive pedagogy aims to embrace diversity and create an environment where all students feel welcome and valued, decolonizing the curriculum actively addresses racism head-on and aims to dismantle racial inequalities in education. Many educators feel that anti-racist pedagogy is contentious because, unlike inclusive pedagogy, which is focused on creating a positive learning environment by valuing diversity, it actively calls out racist narratives, biases, and curriculum omissions by recognizing historical injustices. This means we also focus on challenging racism in our content and integrating diverse perspectives and experiences. On a higher level, it means we critically analyze any power dynamics or institutional biases and take steps to dismantle them.

Key Takeaways:

1. Assist students in developing a "decolonizing attitude" by creating content and learning environments where students who have been historically marginalized are centered and content.

2. The goal of decolonization is to foster inclusive and equitable educational spaces through anti-racist pedagogy by incorporating diverse perspectives, engaging with Indigenous knowledge, challenging dominant narratives, and prioritizing marginalized voices to promote critical thinking, empathy, and social justice in healthcare education.

3. Critically examine the concept of race and its impact on health disparities and gain a deeper understanding of race as a sociopolitical construct that contributes to biases and disparities in health.

CHAPTER 24

•

Sustainability and Metrics for Progress

"What gets counted gets done."
—*Unknown*

Sustainability is imperative for ensuring that inclusion initiatives are authentic, meaningful, and enduring. I firmly believe that just saying we want to foster inclusivity and equity in our institutions is not enough. If we want to transform our culture and climate, we just need to measure our efforts. Similar to the role of data in patient care research, collecting data is instrumental in validating hypotheses related to inclusion and equity in our training programs.

Working with institutions who strive to be more inclusive, I have often heard that we can't measure things like "belonging," or "impact of equity," or "leadership buy-in." And to this, I say, yes, it sometimes takes creativity and long-term vision. We must also ask ourselves other key questions like, *"What are we going to do with the data we are collecting? And how do we know we have met our goals?"* I find the reverse design approach particularly effective in determining the data to collect for equity-driven initiatives. So, imagine if you resolved a major inclusion issue within your organization; what measure would be a clear indication that the issue is no longer an issue? Measuring inclusion and equity through metrics enables us to gain insight into our challenges and gives us direction, hopefully, to address them effectively. It provides a framework to hold stakeholders and leaders accountable for progress while simultaneously facilitating the implementation of targeted interventions to mitigate inequities within our learning environments.

The real challenge is determining *which* metrics to measure and extract that are most relevant amidst so much "noise" in our healthcare and teaching institutions. I believe it starts by adopting a critical mindset and cultivating a heightened awareness of power dynamics in our learning environments. Experimenting with a mixed-method approach allows us to better understand what we want to change in our environment. For example, many institutions have started using pulse surveys to provide a quick read and impression of the educational landscape. These surveys can be valuable for gathering feedback from learners and faculty on specific issues within the curriculum, on campus, or during clerkships. These issues can range from bias and discrimination from preceptors, curricular inclusivity, and systems of support—such as mentorship programs and counseling services—to representation in leadership positions and accessibility. While helpful, if done too often, it can induce survey fatigue and should be attached to transparent messaging of what you will do with the generated data. The data can signal where to start and where to build from and should be considered based on the context in which it is measured to be truly useful.

Let's consider measuring belonging on campus. Some institutions are using tools like the Psychological Sense of School Membership (PSSM) scale, which was first used for adolescent students and later adopted in higher education research. While there isn't a universal instrument that measures belonging in the health sciences, it is worth investigating the Harvard-Panorama Student Perception Survey scale on Sense of Belonging and Yorke's UK-based survey published in 2016 to evaluate student 'belongingness' in higher education.

Interplay of Qualitative and Quantitative Data

In academic medicine, inclusion and culture-related research is often undervalued or dismissed because it may not conform to the familiar scholarly standards associated with clinical research. A shift is needed in our mindsets to recognize that equity and inclusion data is equally potent in propelling cultural change within healthcare training programs. If we are doing inclusion "right," then we are touching these points across multiple aspects of our curricula or operations in higher education. As educators and administrators, we can leverage behavioral measurement approaches, questioning where exclusionary or inequitable outcomes or behaviors exist and understanding their underlying mechanisms. Ultimately, we need measurable changes if we want to see the impact of our efforts and initiatives.

I once heard Brandale Mills Cox, PhD, a quantitative researcher, discuss the "storytelling of data," where both quantitative and qualitative data can show us how the lived experiences of individuals can be looked at through the lens of research insights. We can start with both or one or the other. When analyzing the quantitative or "hard numbers" data, we can determine the correlations to set our inclusion landscape. Qualitative data then provides us with more context to the hard numbers and why they might be landing where they are. While qualitative data can diagnose the problems, gaps, or "whys," quantitative data can paint the storyline around the data. The art of storytelling is really elevated when we use our qualitative data to really tap into emotions and feelings. We can't just rely on quantitative data to inform our strategies toward success.

Let's take a look at how this interplay may look for a medical school that wants to better understand retention patterns and strategies for their students. Diversity prompts us to inquire, "What is the increase in the number of underrepresented students compared to last year?" Equity extends the question to examine, "What choices have we made that keep certain groups as the majority in our program?" Inclusion takes it a step further, asking, "Have we created a welcoming environment that makes everyone feel safe and have a sense of belonging?"

So, a medical school could evaluate diversity by collecting quantitative data on the demographics of admitted students, including information on race, ethnicity, socioeconomic background, and geographic location. They could then analyze this data to identify trends and measure the representation of various groups, emphasizing the representation of underrepresented minority (URM) groups in each incoming class. This data could be assessed to identify any patterns or gaps in retention rates among URM students across each year of the program.

From a qualitative data approach, the school could conduct focus groups and interviews with URM students who have successfully navigated the medical school program longitudinally. These qualitative methods aim to understand if equity and inclusion-based practices are helping contribute to their sense of belonging, academic success, and overall satisfaction. Simultaneously, the program could also interview URM students who may have faced challenges to gather insights into potential barriers. By combining quantitative data with qualitative insights, the medical school gains a nuanced understanding of URM student experiences. The analysis might reveal, for instance, that while there is an increase in URM admissions, there are specific challenges faced during the academic journey. Using this integrated approach, the school can tailor retention strategies that could include mentorship programs, community-building initiatives, or monitoring systems based on both statistical trends and the narratives shared by students.

Case Study: UC Davis School of Medicine's Drive to Diversify Admissions

The medical school at UC Davis is an exemplar of how to diversify a class without relying on race-based criteria. Despite California's prohibition on using race in admissions decisions—enforced since 1996 and reaffirmed by the SCOTUS decision in 2023—the school achieved remarkable diversity in its class of 2026. Notably, outside of HBCUs and Hispanic-serving institutions, UC Davis's class was one of the most diverse in the country, with student demographics including 14% Black, 30% Hispanic, 3% Native American, and 84% from economically disadvantaged backgrounds.

So, how did they do it? Their strategy involved a holistic admissions process that prioritized each candidate's lived experiences beyond traditional metrics like GPA and MCAT scores. The admissions committee introduced multiple mini-interviews, designed to minimize individual bias and better predict future success as a physician. This approach allowed the committee to assess attributes such as maturity, work experience, military service, and personal experiences with illness or disability.

Moreover, UC Davis aligned its admissions goals with the demographics of the communities it serves to enhance provider-patient congruence. By focusing on these diverse aspects of each applicant's background, the school not only addresses state workforce needs but also ensures that the admissions process reflects the varied lived experiences and socioeconomic backgrounds of its applicants.

Leveraging Equity, Inclusion, or Diversity Data Beyond Quotas and Boxes

So, what should we do with the data we generate? Simply filling quotas to address gender, racial, or other representation gaps isn't the end game. We need to use the data as a starting point for the longer journey of retaining the individuals we are trying to recruit. True belonging and inclusion require more than just meeting numerical targets.

When it comes to analyzing data, we can go in many directions. Disaggregating qualitative data can be helpful in determining how gaps and trends appear. For example, how do students from URM groups with disabilities respond compared to those without a disability? Cutting the data in multiple ways can help us better understand our results and come to conclusions about the story. Regression can help confirm new trends.

Critical perspective in data analysis is a way to better understand the nuanced causative factors and broader context in which data was collected and will be used. We have to think about historical power and privilege dynamics when we consider factors that are meeting our academic or admissions standards. What can we do to bring more attention to these inequity gaps? Within higher education or healthcare, we can ask three questions to evaluate the impact of policies or initiatives through the lens of power: 1) Who is benefiting and who is not? Look closely at the distribution of resources, opportunities, and outcomes to discern patterns of advantage and disadvantage. 2) Who made the rules? Examine the composition of decision-making bodies and assess whether diverse perspectives and voices are adequately represented. This can also unveil biases baked into your existing policies or practices. 3) What messages are being used by those who benefit from the current system to maintain the status quo?" Identify what narratives, whether explicit or implicit, are maintaining existing power structures and preventing change.

Filling our representation quotas has lots of baggage around it, and sometimes it can be disadvantageous to BIPOC individuals. When organizations focus solely on meeting representation quotas without addressing the underlying issues of inclusion and equity, it can lead to *tokenism*. We must ask why we want to, for example, "increase the number of faculty or women in our leadership team," and "How we will support them when they join our organization?" This is another space where our quantitative data can help provide some context. The social identity makeup of your student body, faculty, staff, and even the broader community should be simultaneously looked at, while also considering the representation in your administrative team. This allows for diverse perspectives and helps us better align individuals within our classrooms, offices, and clinics. Intersectionality should also be considered when we are analyzing our data. People can fall into multiple categories and experience the world differently. A straight White woman's experience will be very different than that of a non-binary White woman who is disabled.

When we collect participation demographics, we should always offer "prefer to self-describe" open-ended options related to social identities. Relying only on HR or admissions data can be problematic as it can be linked back to employee or student profiles housed by outside vendors or institutions that may not have an equity perspective. We must prioritize participant protection and allow individuals to self-identify whenever possible. This also allows us to evaluate more deeply who is not responding when we have data missing. Looking at gaps in data is also just as important as the data itself. For example, usually, having 10 to 15 people who respond to a question allows for safer data disaggregation, ensuring true anonymity. Another strategy is to broaden your reach and think about other stakeholders like alums, donors, and other communities that also influence your inclusion narrative. One tool that can be used is the "Diversity Index" as a model to assess race, gender, and interprofessional diversity among graduates from health professions schools by benchmarking their distribution to the general population.

Navigating Bias and Humanity in Research

Recognizing the role of the researcher in the research process is also key to data evaluation. We must recognize that we hold biases as researchers who are looking at data. After all, we are human, and perfection is not possible. It is not about impartiality or objectivity but rather about interrupting our implicit biases before analyzing the data. Having a research team with diverse perspectives and social identities helps minimize bias, ensuring all issues are addressed before reaching conclusions. Perfection is often a factor that also comes up. The data generated will never be perfect in an imperfect system or world.

The humanity of the researcher should also be considered when we must navigate "hard to read" data that can be triggering to you as a researcher who might hold marginalized identities. With shared experiences, we can often empathize with the participants' experiences, but as a researcher, this might require some disconnection. For example, creating focus groups by intentionally selecting researchers who will not be harmed by the potential responses of participants is critical. I believe practicing self-care and holding space for our own emotions is critical when we are embarking on social science research.

Key Takeaways:

1. Combine both qualitative and quantitative data to measure the trends and gaps and use them as a starting point to answer deeper questions.

2. Start with the "*why*"—ask why the data is being collected and how it will be used to evaluate the impact of initiatives and measure cultural change.

3. Approaches to inclusion and equity data analysis should move beyond mere representation quotas and consider disaggregating data to explore intersectionality to gain a comprehensive understanding of inequities.

CHAPTER 25

•

Continuing Professional Development

*"Learning is a treasure that will follow
its owner everywhere."*
—Chinese Proverb

Raise your hand if you've been asked by your organization to complete an online module on implicit bias or another diversity, inclusion, and equity-related topic in the past few years. I can imagine most of us chuckling at this because, yes, we have, and we can probably guess how effective that training has been in culture and behavior change. One recurring mistake that health education programs often fall into when striving to establish a fairer and more inclusive learning environment or workplace is focusing on quick wins and then checking the task off as complete. One of those quick wins is often mandating all employees to complete an online training and then calling it a day. I say this safely as someone who has been asked to design and deliver some of these one- to two-hour sessions for many institutions. Even I can see the limitations.

We all have to do mandatory training in all of our jobs, from handling hazardous substances to compliance with HIPAA regulations. Such training does ensure exposure to important standards in our healthcare fields. However, we also know that mandatory training is only step one; we need steps two through 20 to build the stamina of healthcare professionals or educators to change attitudes and behaviors to promote anti-racist and inclusive practices. Also, content can vary widely in quality. With implicit bias, research shows that behaviors don't change with a one-off training module or workshop. It requires building on the knowledge gained and continuously engaging in hands-on applications. Think about this with foundational clinical coursework. We don't expect mastery from our students when we provide an introductory course focused on models of communication to use with patients. It isn't until we provide opportunities to practice models of cross-cultural communication through experiential education and active learning activities like role-playing or simulations that we start to see behavior and attitude change. This moves us past the introduction to reinforcement and mastery. Similarly, the same line of thinking should be applied to professional development related to inclusion. Continuous practice and application drive real, meaningful change.

The other often-asked question that comes up is, "*Should everyone be required to do inclusion or equity-related continuing education?*" To some extent, it is important to fill the knowledge gaps and standardize approaches with a common framework from which we work. On one hand, having mandatory credentialing or training often may not translate to actual change in practice. Just as a healthcare provider attending a continuing education course on diabetes updates doesn't imply they will implement changes to their clinical care—the course still provides valuable guidance about its application. On the other hand, for someone who provides advanced care to patients with diabetes as part of their daily clinical care, this information will feel underwhelming. Furthermore, training that focuses solely on cultural competence may unintentionally influence healthcare professionals to view cultures or identities as static and homogenous, leading to oversimplification and misunderstanding. Promoting cultural humility through ongoing self-reflection and learning can offer a more effective approach, albeit one that is more challenging to implement.

Offering Development Beyond the Human Resources (HR) Modules

I invite you to look at inclusion training and professional development beyond the perspective of stuffy, talk-based lectures, seminars, and workshops focused on topics like stereotyping, anti-racism, or LGBTQ+ affirming care. Think of formats that are not as conventional but allow participants to bring pleasure and joy into connection with one another.

Perhaps you want to offer a retreat or breaks that are designated for exploring art, music, or movement, where people can reconnect to their bodies and passions. Looking at art inspired by various cultural perspectives might not be of interest to everyone, but it provides a point of expanding perspective and building exposure points to "others." Book clubs also foster open discussions across teams and allow a space to explore other's views and insights. Planning a volunteer community service project can be another method to promote engagement and instill social responsibility for others. Consider inviting your residents and students to engage, as well. These various activities are examples of bridging connections through exploring our similarities and differences. They highlight that continuing education in the inclusion realm is not just work but can be based on rest, pleasure, and bonding.

Cultural transformation involves incorporating discussions on health equity and anti-racism into events like grand rounds, case conferences, and medical seminars. Instead of isolated presentations on these topics, they can be integrated into patient case discussions and clinical staff meetings. Racial justice training should encompass a shared language, knowledge, and an understanding of the history of oppression in the United States. It should serve as a platform for sharing, reflection, and mobilization toward institutional change.

Case Study: Filling the Knowledge Gaps

Reflecting on my own experiences of exclusion was crucial in finding solutions for fostering inclusivity at my institution. Like many, I have faced moments of not feeling like I belonged as a student, resident, and professional.

Recognizing that my story was not unique, I felt compelled to honor my heritage of community and collective thought to find a solution. My goal was to inspire faculty and staff to co-create a campus environment centered on empathy and respect for diverse identities and perspectives. This means equipping our faculty and staff with the tools and strategies needed to make our learners feel safe, supported, and empowered to reach their full potential, regardless of their cultural background or identity.

I crafted a proposal, which received approval and funding from my university administration. This initiative led to the creation of a yearlong, two-campus-wide continuing education program designed for faculty and staff across all of our health professions disciplines. The program focused on facilitating authentic and timely discussions about intentional inclusion led by both internal and external subject matter experts.

Each interactive session throughout the year emphasized real-world scenarios, best practices, and actionable steps to enhance interactions with all learners, both inside and outside the classroom. In the planning phase, I drafted the following learning outcomes for participants:

1. Define principles of equity-mindedness, support services, and inclusive teaching.

2. Identify the role of identity and inequities in all learning environments (e.g., classrooms, labs, workshops, etc.).

3. Explain the impact of bias, inequities, and microaggressions on student learning and select appropriate responses in an education setting.

4. Describe effective frameworks, tools, and strategies that promote inclusive practices and environments on campus.

My training in intergroup facilitation (see Chapter 16) allowed me to create a brave and authentic space during our sessions to encourage collaboration and community building so we could better navigate the intricate layers that constitute the fabric of the healthcare academy. Reflecting on the feedback I received following the program's first cohort of graduates, I saw that this provided a much-needed forum to dialogue around the messy day-to-day matters of exclusion, implicit bias, intercultural communication mishaps in the workplace—something a generic HR module could never replace.

Behavior Change and Resources

Beyond providing a structure to professional development, there should also be a focus on measuring the effectiveness of inclusion training. Without data and honest analysis of what the status quo shows us, the outcomes are often limited and fleeting. Although challenging, it is important to assess whether ongoing training efforts lead to meaningful changes in behavior, attitudes, or even patient outcomes in the clinical setting.

Chapter 25

Research shows that just utilizing implicit bias training does very little to change behavior. Jesse Singal's 2023 New York Times opinion piece titled *"What if Diversity Training is Doing More Harm Than Good?"* highlighted that morale from such training can actually take away from interest or commitment to inclusion and equity in an organization. Collecting measurable data, not only recruitment, but retention, satisfaction, and compensation, gives us a better grounding for where we are now and where we are going. Transforming the culture of a hospital or university requires us first to identify the disparities and what fuels them.

Organizations should also allocate sufficient time and resources, including financial and personnel, for comprehensive training if they are genuinely committed to inclusion. The source of training should also be screened so that there isn't inadvertent tokenization of individuals from underrepresented groups as the appointed "experts" on DEI topics. This can not only lead to additional pressure and discomfort for these individuals but also take away from their focus and energy to other career advancements. Content should also be screened to ensure that there isn't unintentional reinforcement of stereotypes or overgeneralized narratives that can perpetuate bias rather than combat it.

Social media can also be a useful resource to leverage. For instance, a 2019 study in the *Journal of Women's Health* found that using Twitter chats to increase awareness of gender equity issues in medicine significantly enhanced the impact of related studies, as indicated by higher Altmetric scores, and led to a notable increase in article downloads and readership. However, for DEI initiatives to effect real behavior and cultural change, organizations and individuals must do more than simply highlight diversity online. It is vital that this visibility is supported by genuine, actionable strategies and a firm commitment to DEI, rather than just engaging in performative actions.

Preventing Burnout for Those Leading Inclusion Work

A cautionary tale of faculty development is that we must be careful that there is no invisible labor put on BIPOC or URM faculty to train others. This can lead to increased burnout and function under the assumption that someone's social identity equates to expertise or comfort in providing professional development. Think about looking outside your department or institution to see if you need to bring in trainers. Also, evaluations of training offered should be considered to provide metrics on what is working and what is not. That "one session or workshop" approach will always fail because repeated actions and time are needed for meaningful and sustainable change. Between these workshops or training sessions, educators and leaders should continue to hold a critical lens to how resources are allocated, policies are developed, and evaluations are performed to ensure that these training events are leading to change toward equity and inclusion.

You miss 100% of the shots you don't take, so don't hesitate to ask for the support you need. This could be resourcing through compensation or financial needs, workforce labor, or even accountability, which ties efforts back to achievable outcomes for your organization's strategic plan.

Many healthcare education organizations have been revising their standards and competencies and creating task forces to work toward dismantling systems of inequity. This involves a continuous effort to address the root causes of health disparities by developing graduates who are culturally sensitive and aware of inequities. Having these standards in place does not replace the real work needed to create a more culturally responsive workforce that starts with faculty and administrative leaders doing the hard work and critical introspection on where they are in the process themselves.

Chapter 25

Key Takeaways:

1. One-off training modules are often ineffective to cultivate inclusive environments. We should shift toward longitudinal and immersive learning experiences to promote greater mastery and application of inclusive practices.

2. Augment traditional methods of continuing education by incorporating bonding and joy-inducing activities like art exploration, music, and community service projects to make inclusion-focused development more engaging and enjoyable.

3. Assessing the impact of inclusion training on behavior, attitudes, and patient outcomes is just as important as allocating sufficient time and resources to professional development.

CHAPTER 26

•

Organizational Culture & Inclusive Leadership

"The ultimate measure of a man is not where he stands in moments of comfort and convenience, but where he stands at times of challenge and controversy."
—Martin Luther King Jr.

In recent years, there has been a surge in the availability of books concentrating on inclusion and organizational culture transformation. While many publications explore the intricacies of organizational leadership, this chapter adopts a unique perspective. Here, our focus shifts toward the need for an inclusive mindset for effective leadership. It's worth noting that in recent times, DEI can also be viewed as limiting, contentious, and even downright polarizing in the workplace. Some touting it as being "too woke" or an agenda for "reverse discrimination." Others focus only on diversity hires and representation as the key fix to all DEI issues. Many others see the role of DEI as a mode to get folks to become more conscious of what is unconscious and put all of their efforts into training and workshops.

While the *whys* and *hows* of DEI at an organizational level differ, what I know to be true across the board is that creating an

Chapter 26

inclusive culture and equitable workplace or learning environment takes time and intentional effort by leaders. I also know that change is hard. *Really hard.*

The saying, "leaders bring the weather," holds significant truth as leaders influence the culture and climate of any organization. By embodying DEI principles, they serve as a model for how team members should engage with others and set standards. This starts with leaders not shying away from centering DEI in their strategic planning, continuous dialogue, and quality-based key performance measures for their organizations. Embracing inclusion requires a willingness to facilitate challenging discussions that redefine power dynamics and a readiness to set and model clear behavioral boundaries. To reinforce equitable practices, we must normalize them in our everyday vernacular. This starts at the top as much as it starts at the grassroots level.

Ingredients for top-down approaches that are often successful amongst healthcare education leaders include engaging in cultural sensitivity and bias training, modeling inclusive behaviors and values, and a commitment to advancing health equity. Leaders must actively speak out and put into writing their program's dedication to anti-oppressive practices, tackling social justice issues within both clinical and educational environments. This commitment helps make invisible issues like structural racism, implicit bias, and unequal care more visible, fostering a culture of accountability. They must also allocate sufficient funding and resources to transform departments and support the objectives of strategic planning.

Investing in inclusion and belonging is a clear reflection of effective leadership. For instance, it is crucial for residency leaders to be actively engaged in this work, considering that residents from underrepresented groups often experience racism and racist incidents in their communities, as we previously discussed in Chapter 15. Faculty and mentors who champion equity and inclusion efforts should be accessible to trainees across all programs, providing a source of validation, support, and sponsorship. Such measures help propel us toward the goal of actively combating racism, sexism, ablest, and other forms of discrimination in healthcare education.

What Makes Inclusive and Equity-minded Leaders?

A couple of years ago, I was asked by a well-known national healthcare academic organization to provide insights into my experiences as an inclusive and equitable leader. I froze while reading the email request to be interviewed. At the time, I didn't have a formal role or title in the DEI space. Why were they asking me? Sure, I had numerous keynote presentations and publications under my belt, and I had been teaching intercultural patient care for over a decade, but I was not a leader in DEI, was I? Being part of this interview and reflecting on my own journey allowed me to realize that leadership is not defined by holding a specific title or role in healthcare or higher education. It is one that is rooted in service and respect, compelling each of us to be inclusive leaders.

As a first-generation American who immigrated to the United States, I had to figure out a lot of things for myself. As a leader, I had the privilege of being guided by mentors invested in building an authentic relationship with me, honoring my Muslim and immigrant roots. These mentors inspired me to uphold my core value of service to students, faculty colleagues, patients, and the profession, even when my perspective diverged from the majority. I now see that being given the breathing room to remain true to my identities and values has played a pivotal role in shaping my success, creating a ripple effect of positive change.

Chapter 26

I see leadership as being about where you want to go and taking people with you regardless of having a formal title or understanding everyone's differences. Inclusive leaders center belonging and know that even if initiatives don't go as planned, they trust themselves enough to know how to respond. For a couple of years, I got to work alongside a White, male Dean of an HBCU on a national grant for the Office of Minority Health, focused on increasing admissions of historically underrepresented minority students. I remember watching him stay quiet for most of our meetings as many of the BIPOC members of the advisory group openly shared their ideas. I felt compelled to ask him after one of our meetings, "What has been your biggest lesson around DEI?" to which he responded, "DEI requires taking baby steps, and I have to keep listening and learning so that I know how to ensure everyone belongs." His deep curiosity not to take up all the airtime and humble servitude showed his willingness to leverage his position to help elicit necessary change. This aligned with what I know is true. Our main metric to know we have succeeded in creating inclusive environments is others' sense of authentic belonging.

Imagine if we measured our success by how safe people felt to be themselves in our presence. One inclusion framework for leaders by Shore and colleagues highlights the delicate balance of belongingness (when one feels they belong to the larger group) and uniqueness (when one's unique qualities are considered important). Inclusion happens when both are high. Assimilation, on the other hand, is when we ignore the differences of individuals and people are forced to "fit in" to be accepted. If actions speak louder than words, and research shows people tend to emulate the behaviors of leaders they respect and trust, what inclusive actions are you modeling to your workforce and learners? How do you show that you value the uniqueness of others?

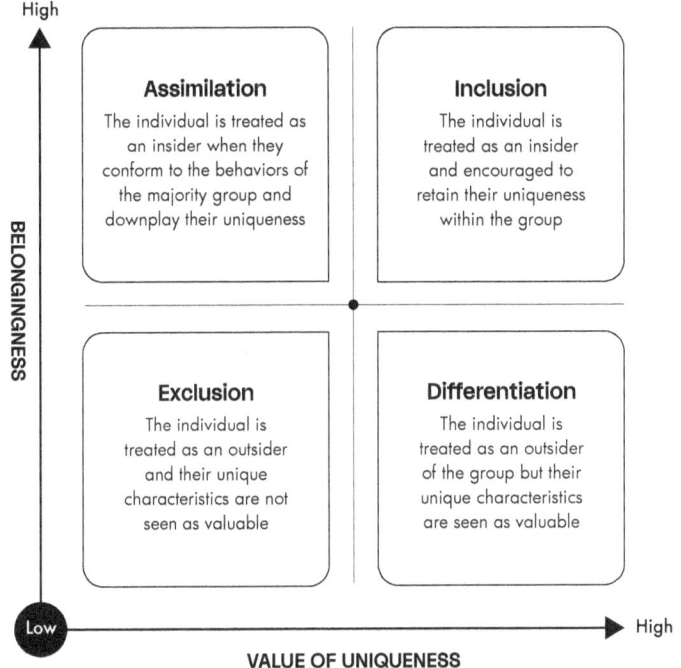

Adapted from: Shore, LM, Randel, AE, Chung, BG. (2011). Inclusion and diversity in work groups: A review and model for future research. *Journal of Management*, 37(4), 1262-1289.

FIGURE 9: INCLUSION FRAMEWORK FOR INDIVIDUALS IN A GROUP

Championing inclusion efforts has made me deeply reflect on my desire to prioritize *psychological safety* as a primary inclusive leadership practice, more so in recent years. My success as a leader is anchored on feedback from learners and colleagues who don't just relay that *"she is motivational and inspiring"* but rather that *"she is empathetic and compassionate to my story."* I often tell the healthcare education administrators I work with as a consultant that we have to start by listening to our most valued assets—our learners and workforce. We must be proactive in requesting feedback from them and truly take in what they have to say with the desire to gain a deeper understanding of the oppressive systems we are aiming to dismantle. This also means doing our homework to gain an understanding of the root issues that create inequities in education and the healthcare system. This is what affords us the opportunity to reflect on and reaffirm why the work we lead matters. If we operate from a 'business case' perspective for inclusion, equity, or diversity, then this will only fuel short-lived change. Rather, we should hold a *social justice* perspective to see long-term, sustainable systemic change. In the spirit of reflecting, as an administrator who wants to grow as an inclusive leader, consider answering these questions:

- What is your unique access to opportunities and resources as a leader? Consider mapping your social identities (see Chapter 7) to evaluate how your privileges and power impact your perceptions, beliefs, behaviors, and responses within your work culture.

- How can you build *brave spaces* to practice facilitating and engaging in successful and difficult conversations across our differences? Creating brave spaces (see Chapter 9) allows for everyone to listen to understand rather than just respond or judge differing opinions or viewpoints. Promoting inclusive meetings, for example, gives everyone the chance to speak without interruption, ask clarifying questions, and validate each other's contributions. Also, consider how comfortable you are conducting dialogues about unconscious bias with peers, managers, and subordinates in order to improve communication and enhance team collaboration.

- Do you invite feedback from your team about your approach toward equity and inclusion? This could be done by asking questions like: What can I do to make you feel more included? How can I create a more inclusive environment where you feel your perspective is as important as mine? How can I better demonstrate my commitment to fostering a culture of inclusion through my actions and decisions?

- How can you develop a more social justice perspective to your vision and plan for an inclusive workplace and team? Take proactive measures to tackle issues such as equitable compensation, impartial promotions, and the establishment of a secure and inclusive work environment. Additionally, demonstrate a commitment to social responsibility and uphold ethical conduct.

Inclusive leaders use both their power and privilege to shift from the "DEI is an HR issue" mindset to "it's a core leadership skill that I need to cultivate within myself." They recognize their privilege and understand that their lived experience is different from those around them. Operating as an advocate means showing solidarity, being willing to take personal risks, and operating with bravery, even when it feels uncomfortable. Inclusive leaders strive to promote psychological safety by making the workplace safer for the team and encouraging them to challenge norms for the sake of a fairer and more just future. Inclusive leaders are not afraid to face pushback when challenging established norms in the pursuit of fairness and equity for all.

Moving Inclusive Leadership from Theory to Practice

"Your present circumstances don't determine where you can go; they merely determine where you start." —Nido Qubein

I remember reading a Harvard Business Review article that cited visible commitment, humility, awareness of bias, curiosity about others, cultural intelligence, and effective collaboration as key traits that inclusive leaders share. While all of these traits resonate with me, I think we have to remember that becoming a truly inclusive leader is a long road. It includes a high tolerance for uncertainty, ambiguity, and difference. We can't just wish inclusion into existence. Inclusive leaders embrace and anticipate push-back when disrupting the status quo, recognizing it as a natural part of driving meaningful change.

Cultural humility involves understanding the complexity of identities, beliefs, practices, and cultural values of diverse populations and recognizing our own biases and prejudices. So, when I practice inclusive leadership, I need to have the ability to manage a diverse group of people while respecting their unique characteristics. This means ensuring that everyone has the opportunity to contribute to discussions and decision-making, regardless of their backgrounds. This also means that accessing information and advancement is not a barrier. For instance, requesting that all video meetings be closed-captioned and actively advocating for diverse representation in leadership roles within your organization.

Feedback is a gift for action. Supervisors and leaders, as allies, should be aware of their responsibility to take additional steps if an individual reveals harassment or discrimination concerns. Express gratitude for their openness and trust in sharing information, and acknowledge the bravery it takes to come forward. It's also important to inquire about their preferences regarding any actions you should take based on the disclosed information. Demonstrate active listening and inquire if they are open to providing additional clarification if needed. If a concern constitutes a legal violation or policy breach, it is advisable to communicate any obligations to disclose or report specific information to them before they articulate their concerns. This proactive approach empowers individuals to make informed choices about the information they choose to share.

Furthermore being aware of our own implicit biases requires that we proactively seek out different viewpoints that inform better decisions for our learners, colleagues, patients, and community. Outside of work, try to seek opportunities to engage with individuals or groups who are different from you to broaden your understanding of others. Actively pursuing an understanding of diverse cultural norms and perspectives helps develop our *cultural intelligence.* By doing so, we can better adapt our behaviors and mindsets to navigate cross-cultural interactions and lead more effectively.

On a systemic level, moving DEI efforts from theory to practice should always start with creating a clear and thoughtful strategic plan and timeline with opportunities for feedback. Methods should be in place for how actions and plans will be executed and assessed. This sends a beacon to your learners and faculty community that you are not check-boxing your way to equity and inclusion. Listening and dialogue sessions with stakeholders should conclude with a clear outline of how the discussed values will be implemented into practice. This ensures that equity-minded principles are consistently integrated into the organization's decision-making processes and everyday practices.

For leaders who appreciate organized frameworks, here are essential components for advancing inclusion efforts and ensuring their successful implementation. Utilize this list as a screening tool to assess your progress and identify areas for further advancement:

- **Ensure commitment to outcomes:** Emphasize both enthusiasm and commitment to inclusion goals within your organization.
- **Collect and track diversity data:** Gather accurate data on faculty and trainees in key departmental segments (e.g., divisions, residency program, and fellowship programs).

- **Set specific goals:** Establish clear objectives for increased diversity and inclusion that consider key demographic characteristics and goals for advancement, such as promotions and leadership roles.

- **Implement and evaluate programmatic strategies:** Develop and execute specific strategies to achieve diversity and inclusion goals, which are regularly assessed for effectiveness. This could include the effectiveness of continuing professional development for your workforce.

- **Provide sufficient funding:** Allocate the necessary resources and investment to support culture transformation efforts. What do other divisions of your program get? Are you willing to give the same for your inclusion initiatives to get the same for them to also thrive and succeed?

- **Track intervention outcomes:** Monitor and measure the outcomes resulting from implemented interventions by analyzing the data to assess progress and identify areas for improvement.

- **Continuously improve interventions:** Utilize feedback and effectiveness evaluations to enhance and update interventions. Don't be afraid to make necessary adjustments to optimize outcomes. Pivoting is part of the game!

- **Designate a responsible and accountable leader:** Appoint a senior leader with authority, influence, and resources to oversee outcomes linked to representation, inclusion, and equity.

- **Incentivize leadership prioritization:** Encourage other leaders to prioritize and actively contribute to inclusion efforts. This is everyone's responsibility, and there should be incentives and recognition for making tangible progress in DEI.

Overcoming Challenges

Incorporating inclusivity into our institution comes with its share of hurdles, but there are also effective strategies we can use to address them. We must start by seeing the whole picture and not just focusing on what we know. This means becoming curious about how our policies and procedures might contribute to inequities for our learners and workforce.

We often operate by creating SMART goals in our policy and practice building (**S**pecific, **M**easurable, **A**ctionable, **R**easonable, and **T**ime-bound) but don't center equity and inclusion in our goal setting and our processes. I have found moving to a SMARTIE goal where we integrate "IE" after SMART which stands for Inclusive and Equitable. This helps us create educational equity a reality for ALL—whether this is in how we address salary inequities, conduct our pharmacy candidate interviews, or provide accommodations to students, we are better able to affirm and keep ourselves accountable to our core value of inclusion.

We also have to reflect the communities we serve, which means we have to look at who is being represented in our leadership. One of our deficiencies in healthcare leadership is that we don't see what we are missing, and the service mission that we provide does not stop with the students and patients in our institutions but extends to engaging with the community.

Another challenge is that DEI initiatives are often checkboxed or siloed rather than being created as part of an institution or program's strategic plan. So there is a built-in blueprint for change and accountability so that efforts are sustainable. Inclusion and equity goal setting should never be as a "one and done" project or given to just one volunteer-based ad hoc committee to complete or be accountable for.

Embracing Emotional Intelligence

Conflict, misunderstandings, and disagreements are expected in healthcare settings and health professions programs. When leaders react to these moments with defense or dismiss concerns, they send a clear message that they are not able to connect to the emotional needs of their learners or workforce. There hasn't been a clearer reason for the exit from an institution of higher learning or healthcare that can't be linked back to some degree of lack of emotional intelligence by its leaders. It erodes trust and creates an environment where the workforce feels unvalued and unsupported, especially when they already hold underrepresented and misunderstood identities.

In order to implement and promote inclusive practices, we need to integrate the key ingredient of emotional intelligence. A concept introduced in the 1990s by social scientists Peter Salovey and John Mayer, emotional intelligence is defined as "the ability to monitor one's own and others' feelings and emotions, to discriminate among them, and use this information to guide thinking and actions. This includes characteristics like advocacy, social skills, brave leadership, self-awareness, and empathy, which, as a leader, are inherently important. Inclusive leaders demonstrate a strong ability to understand and empathize with the perspectives, feelings, and experiences of their workforce, especially when they come from diverse backgrounds or circumstances. Leaders with emotional intelligence actively seek to understand the unique challenges faced by others and role model what it means to not react to problems but rationally and sensitively respond to them. Developing emotional intelligence is an ongoing process that requires returning to the practice of cultural humility and maintaining a willingness to learn and improve, regardless of one's rank, title, or experience in their role. An unchecked ego suffocates cultural humility.

Impactful leadership demands introspection. To help you deepen your emotional self-awareness, consider these reflective questions:

- How do you effectively manage your emotions, especially in challenging or uncertain situations, to set a positive example for your team?
- How aware are you of the emotions and moods of your team, and what evidence do you have for this?
- How do you actively seek and consider their perspectives and feelings? In what ways do you foster an inclusive and emotionally supportive environment where team members feel comfortable expressing themselves?

Key Takeaways:

1. Creating inclusive cultures and equitable workplaces takes time, intentional effort, and facing challenges.

2. Leaders set the tone and play a crucial role in shaping organizational culture. This means leadership should embrace emotional intelligence as they aim to embody inclusive practices and actively integrate them into strategic planning and key performance measures.

3. Challenge the notion that inclusive leadership is solely based on formal roles or titles, but rather, based on serving and respect where psychological safety, authentic belonging, and actively listening to stakeholders are prioritized.

APPENDIX

Book Discussion Guide

(...because authors shouldn't have the last word!)

The world changes one conversation at a time, and each reader has a unique perspective to bring to the table. Here are some questions to get your dialogue going with others after reading this book:

1. What parts of the historical context of inequities in higher education or healthcare have been most surprising to learn about? How does understanding this context help inform and shape your approach to teaching, research, service, or leadership going forward?

2. How has doing your own social identity mapping shifted the way you view and engage with inclusion efforts? If you haven't done any social identity exploration, what do you feel is holding you back?

3. Which principles outlined in the book resonated most with you? Why?

4. How has engaging with the SHIFT framework changed your experiences on campus, in the healthcare setting, or in your personal life?

5. Describe a time you have seen allyship not work. What lessons did you learn from this instance, and how could it have been more effective?

6. In what ways can we prioritize connection over content in our health education settings? What are the barriers to this at your institution?

7. Which practices of integrating inclusion and equity into teaching, scholarship, or patient care are already happening around you? Which are not? What do you feel is driving both?

8. Where do you still have discomfort or resistance as you read through the principles and areas of practice? Name these and reflect on what might be driving your feelings.

9. What is one way you can disrupt your teaching or mentoring practices to be more equitable or inclusive based on the strategies given in the practice chapters?

10. What are ways your institution can expand its organizational culture to include more diversity, inclusion, or equity-driven strategies? As a leader, where can you push past your comfort zone to embrace more inclusive practices?

Glossary

This **glossary** is not intended to be an exhaustive list of every word and term used in advancing diversity, equity, inclusion, and social justice. These are basic working definitions to be used as a reference to begin important conversations. Here is a friendly reminder that the lexicon will continue to evolve so keep striving to learn!

- **Ally:** A person of one social identity group who stands up in support of members of another group.
- **Anti-racism:** The practice of identifying, challenging, and changing values, structures, and behaviors that perpetuate systemic racism.
- **Belonging:** A sentiment or feeling of connectedness that all people can thrive in and be valued and accepted, which is reinforced by the organization's culture.
- **BIPOC:** Black, Indigenous, (and) People of Color
- **Brave space**: An environment where individuals are encouraged to engage in open, honest, and challenging conversations, with a focus on learning, growth, and mutual respect.
- **Cultural Humility**: A lifelong commitment and practice of self-evaluation and self-critique. This includes examining one's own beliefs, biases, and power imbalances while learning about and respecting others' cultures.
- **Decolonize:** The deliberate and proactive process of shedding values, beliefs, and notions that have inflicted physical, emotional, or mental harm on individuals due

to colonization, necessitating an acknowledgment of oppressive systems.

- **Diversity:** The wide variety of shared and different personal and group characteristics among human beings that is seen as a representation often across social identity lines (e.g., race, gender, age, ability, etc.).
- **Equality:** A state of affairs in which all people within a specific society have the same status, rights, and access.
- **Equity:** The fair treatment, access, resources, and opportunities for all people. Equity considers social identifiers (i.e., race, socioeconomic status, etc.) faced with inequalities needing to be overcome.
- **Inclusive Language:** Refers to language that "includes" all persons in its references.
- **Inclusion:** Creating through action environments that authentically brings traditionally excluded individuals and/or groups into processes, activities, and decision/policy making in a way that shares power.
- **Integration:** Incorporation of individuals or groups into different groups, societies, or organizations as equals.
- **Justice:** Entails fair and equitable access to power, ensuring effectiveness, accountability, and inclusivity at all levels, while simultaneously dismantling barriers to resources and opportunities in society to enable all individuals and communities to lead a full and dignified life.
- **Liberation**: Practices that dismantle the source(s) of inequity. Living with no barriers.
- **Psychological Safety**: Creating an environment where individuals feel comfortable sharing ideas, speaking up

candidly, making mistakes, and taking risks without fear of retaliation, criticism, or ridicule.
- **Solidarity**: Unity and mutual support among individuals or groups, especially during challenges through action.
- **Structural Humility**: Recognizing and addressing the systemic and institutional dimensions that uphold inequities to foster more equitable and inclusive environments. Requires health providers to not be complicit in the inequitable systems they work in.
- **Tolerance**: Acceptance and open-mindedness to different practices, attitudes, and cultures; does not require agreement with the differences.

Barriers to Inclusion and Equity

- **Ableism**: Prejudiced/discriminatory thoughts/actions against individuals with a disability inferring they are inferior to individuals without a disability.
- **Ageism**: Prejudiced/discriminatory thoughts/actions based on age.
- **Classism**: Prejudiced thoughts and discriminatory actions based on a difference in socioeconomic status.
- **Cultural Taxation**: The responsibility imposed on individuals with marginalized identities to educate others about their culture, experiences, and perspectives, frequently without receiving proper compensation or acknowledgment. Sometimes referred to as the "minority tax or burden."
- **Discrimination**: Denial of fair treatment by both individuals and institutions on the basis of a social identity.

- **Implicit/Unconscious Bias**: Negative associations expressed habitually that people unknowingly hold and that affect understanding, actions, and decisions; also known as unconscious or hidden bias.

- **Intersectionality**: An approach arguing that classifications cannot be examined in isolation from one another; rather, intersecting in individuals' lives, society, social systems, and are mutually constitutive. A social construct acknowledging the fluid diversity of identities individuals can hold, encompassing factors like gender, race, class, religion, professional status, marital status, socioeconomic status, etc.

- **Microaggressions**: The way in which unconscious bias shows up in everyday behavior. Microaggressions may be intentional or unintentional way of communicating through verbal or behavioral actions that land as a prejudiced insult toward a marginalized group. A form of subtle discrimination that is as harmful to a person's physical and psychological well-being as explicit discrimination.

- **Marginalized/Minoritized**: Refers to individuals or groups pushed to society's margins due to factors beyond one's control. This term applies to those outside the dominant group who, despite not being a numerical minority, face systemic disadvantages and are considered minoritized.

- **Oppression**: The pervasive and systemic presence of social inequality extending across societal institutions and individual awareness. Intersects institutional and systemic discrimination with personal bias, bigotry, and social prejudice, creating intricate connections within relationships and structures.

- **Other/othering**: A phenomenon where certain individuals or groups are not treated as they are part of a group because they don't conform to the norms of a social group.
- **Prejudice**: A set of [usually] negative personal beliefs about a social group that leads individuals to prejudge members from that group or the group in general, regardless of discrete differences among members of that group.
- **Privilege**: Unearned access to resources, or social power, only readily available to some individuals as a result of their social group.
- **Stereotype**: Blanket beliefs and expectations about members of certain groups that present an oversimplified opinion or uncritical judgment. *Stereotype threat* is when an individual internalizes negative stereotypes about their social group, which can undermine academic outcomes, performance, and confidence.
- **Tokenism**: The practice of including individuals from underrepresented backgrounds in a setting to create an appearance of diversity without affording them genuine influence or equal opportunities.
- **White Supremacy Culture**: An ideology and set of practices that maintain and prioritize "whiteness" as dominant, "correct," and more valued than other racial and ethnic groups.
- **Xenophobia**: Hatred or fear of foreigners/strangers or of their politics or culture.

Notes

Chapter 1. How We Got Here

- Devakumar, D., Selvarajah, S., Abubakar, I., Kim, S.-S., McKee, M., Sabharwal, N. S., Saini, A., Shannon, G., White, A. I. R., & Achiume, E. T. (2022). Racism, xenophobia, discrimination, and the determination of health. *The Lancet*, 400(10368), 2097–2108.
- Haider, A. H., Weygandt, P. L., Bentley, J. M., Monn, M. F., Rehman, K. A., Zarzaur, B. L., Crandall, M. L., Cornwell, E. E., & Cooper, L. A. (2013). Disparities in trauma care and outcomes in the United States. *Journal of Trauma and Acute Care Surgery*, 74(5), 1195–1205.
- Schulman, K. A., Berlin, J. A., Harless, W., Kerner, J. F., Sistrunk, S., Gersh, B. J., Dubé, R., Taleghani, C. K., Burke, J. E., Williams, S., Eisenberg, J. M., Ayers, W., & Escarce, J. J. (1999). The Effect of Race and Sex on Physicians' Recommendations for Cardiac Catheterization. *New England Journal of Medicine*, 340(8), 618–626.
- Smedley, B. D., Stith, A. Y., & Nelson, A. R. (2003). *Unequal Treatment*. National Academies Press.

Chapter 2. Historical Context and Persisting Barriers

- Alsan, M., & Wanamaker, M. (2018). Tuskegee and the Health of Black Men. *The Quarterly Journal of Economics*, 133(1), 407–455.
- Devakumar, D., Selvarajah, S., Abubakar, I., Kim, S.-S., McKee, M., Sabharwal, N. S., Saini, A., Shannon, G., White, A. I. R., & Achiume, E. T. (2022). Racism, xenophobia, discrimination, and the determination of health. *The Lancet*, 400(10368), 2097–2108.
- Khan, F. A. (2011). The immortal life of Henrietta Lacks. *Journal of the Islamic Medical Association of North America*, 43(2), 93–94.
- King, T. E., Wheeler, M. B., Fernandez, A., Schillinger, D., Bindman, A. B., Grumbach, K., & Villela, T. J. (2006). *Medical Management of Vulnerable & Underserved Patients: Principles, Practice, Population*. McGraw Hill Professional.
- National Human Genome Research Institute. (2022, May 18). *Eugenics and Scientific Racism*.
- Office of Disease Prevention and Health Promotion. (2022, February 6). *Healthy People 2020 Disparities Data*.
- Tervalon, M., & Murray-García, J. (1998). Cultural Humility Versus Cultural Competence: A Critical Distinction in Defining Physician Training Outcomes in Multicultural Education. *J Health Care Poor Underserved*, 9(2), 117–125.

- U.S. Department of Health & Human Services. (n.d.). *CLAS Standards.* Think Cultural Health.
- Victor, R. G., Lynch, K., Li, N., Blyler, C., Muhammad, E., Handler, J., Brettler, J., Rashid, M., Hsu, B., Foxx-Drew, D., Moy, N., Reid, A. E., & Elashoff, R. M. (2018). A Cluster-Randomized Trial of Blood-Pressure Reduction in Black Barbershops. *New England Journal of Medicine, 378*(14), 1291–1301.

Chapter 3. Diversity & Access Laws in Higher Education

- Barnes, R. (2023, June 27). How Supreme Court ruled on affirmative action in the past. *Washington Post*; The Washington Post.
- Bleemer, Z. (2023). Affirmative action and its race-neutral alternatives. *Journal of Public Economics, 220*, 104839.
- Campbell, H. E., Hagan, A. M., Hincapie, A. L., Gaither, C., Freeman, M. K., & Avant, N. D. (2020). Racial disproportionality of students in United States colleges of pharmacy. *Currents in Pharmacy Teaching and Learning, 12*(5), 524–530.
- Capers, Q., Clinchot, D., McDougle, L., & Greenwald, A. G. (2017). Implicit Racial Bias in Medical School Admissions. *Academic Medicine, 92*(3), 365–369.
- Reynolds, A., & Lewis, D. (2017, March 30). *Teams Solve Problems Faster When They're More Cognitively Diverse.* Harvard Business Review.
- Salsberg, E., Brantley, E., Westergaard, S., Farrell, J., & Rosenthal, C. (2021). Limited, uneven progress in increasing racial and ethnic diversity of dental school graduates. *Journal of Dental Education, 86*(1).
- Shen, M. J., Peterson, E. B., Costas-Muñiz, R., Hernandez, M. H., Jewell, S. T., Matsoukas, K., & Bylund, C. L. (2017). The Effects of Race and Racial Concordance on Patient-Physician Communication: A Systematic Review of the Literature. *Journal of Racial and Ethnic Health Disparities, 5*(1), 117–140.
- Smedley, B. D., Adrienne Stith Butler, Bristow, L. R., Institute Of Medicine (U.S.). Committee On Institutional And Policy-Level Strategies For Increasing The Diversity Of The U.S. Health Care Workforce, & Institute Of Medicine (U.S.). Board On Health Sciences Policy. (2004). *In the nation's compelling interest : ensuring diversity in the health-care workforce.* National Academies Press.

Chapter 4. The Language and Frameworks of Inclusion

- CAST. (2018). *Universal Design for Learning Guidelines.* Cast.org. http://udlguidelines.cast.org
- Center for Urban Education. (n.d.). *CUE Racial Equity Tools.* CUE Racial Equity Tools.
- Columbia Center for Teaching and Learning. (2021). *Teaching in Times of Stress and Challenge.* Columbia University.

- Dias-Broens, A. S., Meeuwisse, M., & Severiens, S. E. (2024). The definition and measurement of sense of belonging in higher education: A systematic literature review with a special focus on students' ethnicity and generation status in higher education. *Educational Research Review, 45*(100622).
- Hanauer, D. I., Graham, M. J., & Hatfull, G. F. (2016). A Measure of College Student Persistence in the Sciences (PITS). *CBE—Life Sciences Education, 15*(4), ar54.
- Malik, L. (2021, June 3). *A "Belongingness" Framework for your Diversity, Equity, and Inclusion Journey*. Thought Ensemble.
- Myers, V. (2015). Diversity is Being Invited to the Party: Inclusion is Being Asked to Dance [Video]. In *AppNexus' inaugural Women's Leadership Forum*.
- Nakintu, S. (2021, November 29). *Diversity, Equity and Inclusion: Key Terms and Definitions*. NACo.
- Paris, D., & Alim, H. S. (2017). *Culturally Sustaining Pedagogies: Teaching and Learning for Justice in a Changing World* (pp. 1–21). Teachers College Press.

Chapter 5. Cycles of Socialization and Narratives

- Adams, M. (2000). *Readings for Diversity and Social Justice: an Anthology on Racism, Antisemitism, Sexism, Heterosexism, Ableism, and Classism* (1st ed., pp. 15–21). Routledge.
- Douglas, A. V. A. (2019, August 22). *Applying Counter-Narratives to Academic Librarianship*. ACRLog.
- Harro, B. (2000). The Cycle of Socialization. In *National Education Association* (pp. 1–9). National Education Association.
- Hobbs, R. (2011). *Digital and Media Literacy: Connecting Culture and Classroom*. Corwin Press.
- Hylton, R. (2022). Using counter-narrative to disrupt dominant perspectives in education: An exploration of the pedagogy and positionality of selected black women faculty. *Journal of Curriculum and Pedagogy*, 1–23.
- Jenkins, H., & Carpentier, N. (2013). Theorizing participatory intensities. *Convergence: The International Journal of Research into New Media Technologies, 19*(3), 265–286.
- Miller, R., Liu, K., & Ball, A. F. (2020). Critical Counter-Narrative as Transformative Methodology for Educational Equity. *Review of Research in Education, 44*(1), 269–300.
- Prilleltensky, I. (2020, July 21). *Challenging Oppressive Narratives | Office of Institutional Culture | University of Miami*. Culture.miami.edu

Chapter 6. The SHIFT Framework

- AAPA. (2013). *Guidelines for Ethical Conduct for the PA Profession*.

- American Academy of Physician Associates. (2021). 2021-2025 Strategic Plan. In www.aapa.org.
- American Pharmacists Association. (2021, November). *Oath of a Pharmacist*. Pharmacist.com.
- Diversity and Inclusion | *American Dental Association*. (n.d.). www.ada.org.
- McGowan, M. (2021, March 1). *What If Doctors Were Paid to Keep People Well?* Center for Nutrition Studies.
- North, M. (2012, February 7). *Greek Medicine - the Hippocratic Oath*. Nih.gov; U.S. National Library of Medicine.
- NOVA | Doctors' Diaries | *The Hippocratic Oath: Modern Version* | PBS. (n.d.). www.pbs.org

Chapter 7. Self-Reflect Critically

- Allison, R., & Banerjee, P. (2014). Intersectionality and Social Location in Organization Studies, 1990-2009. *Race, Gender & Class, 21*(3/4), 67–87.
- Crenshaw, K. (1989). Demarginalizing the Intersection of Race and Sex: a Black Feminist Critique of Antidiscrimination Doctrine, Feminist Theory and Antiracist Politics. *University of Chicago Legal Forum, 1989*(1), 139–167.
- Department of Psychology, & Stanford University. (n.d.). *Map Your Identities | SPARQtools*. Sparqtools.org; Stanford University.
- Hogg, M. A., & Abrams, D. (1990). Social Motivation, Self-Esteem and Social Identity. In Social Identity Theory: Constructive and Critical Advances (pp. 28–47). London: Harvester Wheatsheaf.

Chapter 8. Honor Cultural and Structural Humility

- Assemi, M., Mutha, S., & Hudmon, K. S. (2007). Evaluation of a Train-the-Trainer Program for Cultural Competence. *American Journal of Pharmaceutical Education, 71*(6), 110.
- Cobb, J. (2021, September 10). *The Man Behind Critical Race Theory*. The New Yorker.
- Collins, S. L., Smith, T. C., Hack, G., & Moorhouse, M. D. (2023). Exploring public health education's integration of critical race theories: A scoping review. *Frontiers in Public Health*, 11.
- Crenshaw, K., Gotanda, N., Peller, G., & Thomas, K. (1995). *Critical race theory: the key writings that formed the movement*. The New Press.
- Ford, C. L., & Airhihenbuwa, C. O. (2010). Critical Race Theory, Race Equity, and Public Health: Toward Antiracism Praxis. *American Journal of Public Health, 100*(S1), S30–S35.

- Ford, C. L., & Airhihenbuwa, C. O. (2018). Commentary: Just What is Critical Race Theory and What's it Doing in a Progressive Field like Public Health? *Ethnicity and Disease, 28*(Supp 1), 223.
- Freire, P., Ramos, M. B., & Macedo, D. P. (2014). *Pedagogy of the oppressed.* Bloomsbury Academic.
- Grauf-Grounds, C., Sellers, T. S., Edwards, S. A., Cheon, H.-S., MacDonald, D., Whitney, S., & Rivera, P. M. (2020). A Practice Beyond Cultural Humility. In *Routledge eBooks* (1st ed.). Routledge.
- Hayes, B. (2008). Increasing the Representation of Underrepresented Minority Groups in US Colleges and Schools of Pharmacy. *American Journal of Pharmaceutical Education, 72*(1), 14.
- Irfan, M., Saleem, U., Sethi, M. R., & Abdullah, A. S. (2019). Do We Need To Care: Emotional Intelligence And Empathy Of Medical And Dental Students. *Journal of Ayub Medical College Abbottabad, 31*(1), 76–81.
- Ladson-Billings, G. (1995). But that's just good teaching! The case for culturally relevant pedagogy. *Theory into Practice, 34*(3), 159–165.
- Mantzourani, E. (Efthymia), Courtier, N., Davies, S., & Bean, G. (2015). Perceptions of faculty in health care and social sciences on teaching international students. *Currents in Pharmacy Teaching and Learning, 7*(5), 635–644.
- Rockich-Winston, N., & Wyatt, T. R. (2019). The Case for Culturally Responsive Teaching in Pharmacy Curricula. *American Journal of Pharmaceutical Education, 83*(8), 7425.
- Smedley, B. D. (2012). The Lived Experience of Race and Its Health Consequences. *American Journal of Public Health, 102*(5), 933–935.
- Tsai, J., Lindo, E., & Bridges, K. (2021). Seeing the Window, Finding the Spider: Applying Critical Race Theory to Medical Education to Make Up Where Biomedical Models and Social Determinants of Health Curricula Fall Short. *Frontiers in Public Health,* 9.
- Zaidi, Z., Vyas, R., Verstegen, D., Morahan, P., & Dornan, T. (2017). Medical Education to Enhance Critical Consciousness. *Academic Medicine, 92*(11S Association of American Medical Colleges Learn Serve Lead: Proceedings of the 56th Annual Research in Medical Education Sessions), S93–S99.

Chapter 9. Invite Vulnerability and Discomfort

- Arao, B., & Clemens, K. (2013). From safe spaces to brave spaces: A new way to frame dialogue around diversity and social justice. In L. M. Landreman (Ed.), *The art of effective facilitation: Reflections from social justice educators* (1st ed., pp. 135–150). Routledge.
- Bullough, R. (2005). Teacher Vulnerability and Teachability: A Case Study of a Mentor and Two Interns. *Teacher Education Quarterly, 32*(2).

- Hammond, Z. L. (2014). *Culturally Responsive Teaching and the Brain.* SAGE Publications.
- Wolbring, G., & Lillywhite, A. (2023). Burnout through the Lenses of Equity/Equality, Diversity and Inclusion and Disabled People: A Scoping Review. *Societies, 13*(5), 131.

Chapter 10. Foster Connection Over Content

- Grover, N. (2021, October 7). *Teaching and Learning with Compassion | Harvard Graduate School of Education.* www.gse.harvard.edu.
- Hockings C. (2010). *Inclusive Learning and Teaching in Higher Education: A Synthesis of Research.* Higher Education Academy, York.
- Hockings, C., Brett, P., & Terentjevs, M. (2012). Making a difference—inclusive learning and teaching in higher education through open educational resources. *Distance Education, 33*(2), 237–252.
- Hughes, K., Corcoran, T., & Slee, R. (2015). Health-inclusive higher education: listening to students with disabilities or chronic illnesses. *Higher Education Research & Development, 35*(3), 488–501.
- Moriña, A., Cortés-Vega, M. D., & Molina, V. M. (2015). Faculty training: an unavoidable requirement for approaching more inclusive university classrooms. *Teaching in Higher Education, 20*(8), 795–806.

Chapter 11. Think Active Allyship

- Arif, S., Afolabi, T., Mitrzyk, B. M., Thomas, T. F., Borja-Hart, N., Wade, L., & Henson, B. (2021). Engaging in Authentic Allyship as Part of Our Professional Development. *American Journal of Pharmaceutical Education, 86*(5), 8690.
- Bishop, A. (2015). *Becoming an ally : breaking the cycle of oppression in people.* Fernwood.
- Dainkeh, F. (2019, November 14). *Understanding Intent vs Impact.* She+ Geeks Out.
- Edwards, K. E. (2007). Aspiring Social Justice Ally Identity Development: A Conceptual Model. *NASPA Journal, 43*(4).
- Freire, P. (1970). *Pedagogy of the Oppressed.* Penguin Books.
- Long, S. (2020, May 28). *The Black Community Needs Stronger White Allies — Here's How You Can Be One.* www.refinery29.com.
- Luke, D. J. (2022, April 21). *Ways to Incorporate DEI into Your Courses.* Sage College DEI — Open Dialogue; SAGE Publications Inc.
- Luthra, P. (2022). *The Art of Active Allyship.* Talented Consultancy APS.
- Nixon, S. A. (2019). The coin model of privilege and critical allyship: implications for health. *BMC Public Health, 19*(1).

- Spanierman, L. B., & Smith, L. (2017). Roles and Responsibilities of White Allies: Implications for Research, Teaching, and Practice. *Counseling Psychology*, *45*(5), 606–617.

Chapter 12. Moving Principles into Action

- Carethers, J. M. (2020). Toward realizing diversity in academic medicine. *Journal of Clinical Investigation*, *130*(11), 5626–5628.
- Smith, D. G. (2012). Building Institutional Capacity for Diversity and Inclusion in Academic Medicine. *Academic Medicine*, *87*(11), 1511–1515.

Chapter 13. Intentional Course Design

- Fritzgerald, A. & Rice, S. (2020). *Antiracism and universal design for learning : building expressways to success*. Cast Professional Publishing, An Imprint Of Cast, Inc.
- Charon, R. (2001). Narrative medicine: a model for empathy, reflection, profession, and trust. *JAMA*, *286*(15), 1897.
- Chardin, M. & Novak, K. (2020). *Equity by Design*. Corwin.
- Rolfe, G., Freshwater, D., & Jasper, M. (2001). *Critical Reflection for Nursing and the Helping Professions: A User's Guide*. Palgrave Macmillan.
- Sandars, J. (2009). The use of reflection in medical education: AMEE Guide No. 44. *Medical Teacher*, *31*(8), 685–695.
- Tanner, K. D. (2020). Structure matters: Twenty-One teaching strategies to promote student engagement and cultivate classroom equity. *CBE—Life Sciences Education*, *12*(3), 322–331

Chapter 14. Equity-Minded Syllabus Development

- Baecker, D. L. (1998). Uncovering the Rhetoric of the Syllabus: The Case of the Missing I. *College Teaching*, *46*(2), 58–62.
- Covington, M., Chavis, T., & Perry, A. (2017). A scholar-practitioner perspective to promoting minority success in STEM. *Journal of Multicultural Education*, *11*(2), 149–159.
- Harnish, R. J., & Bridges, K. R. (2011). Effect of syllabus tone: students' perceptions of instructor and course. *Social Psychology of Education*, *14*(3), 319–330. https://doi.org/10.1007/s11218-011-9152-4
- Roberts, M. T. (n.d.). *Syllabus Review Guide*. Center for Urban Education, University of Southern California.
- Taylor, S. D., Veri, M. J., Eliason, M., Hermoso, J. C. R., Bolter, N. D., & Van Olphen, J. E. (2019). The Social Justice Syllabus Design Tool. *Journal Committed to Social Change on Race and Ethnicity*, *5*(2), 133-166.

Chapter 15. Equity-Minded Assessments

- Bali, M., & Zamora, M. (2022). The Equity-Care Matrix: Theory and Practice. *Italian Journal of Educational Technology, 30*(1).
- Capper, G. (2022, February 15). *Belonging inclusion and mental health are all connected.* Wonkhe. https://wonkhe.com/blogs/belonging-inclusion-and-mental-health-are-all-connected
- Denial, C. (2019, August 15). *A Pedagogy of Kindness.* Hybrid Pedagogy.
- Eddy, S. L., & Hogan, K. A. (2014). Getting Under the Hood: How and for Whom Does Increasing Course Structure Work? *CBE—Life Sciences Education, 13*(3), 453–468.
- Gachago, D., Bali, M., & Pallitt, N. (2022). Compassionate Learning Design as a Critical Approach to Instructional Design. In *Toward a Critical Instructional Design.* Hybrid Pedagogy Inc.
- General Pharmaceutical Council. (2021). *Standards for the initial education and training of pharmacists.*
- Gorny-Wegrzyn, E., & Perry, B. (2021). Inspiring Educators and a Pedagogy of Kindness: A Reflective Essay. *Creative Education, 12*(01), 220–230.
- Howansky, K., Maimon, M., & Sanchez, D. (2021). Identity Safety Cues Predict Instructor Impressions, Belonging, and Absences in the Psychology Classroom. *Teaching of Psychology, 49*(3), 009862832199036.
- Jazaieri, H. (2018). Compassionate education from preschool to graduate school. *Journal of Research in Innovative Teaching & Learning, 11*(1), 22–66.
- Koutselini, M. (2017). The Reflective Paradigm in Higher Education and Research: Compassion in Communities of Learning. In *The Pedagogy of Compassion at the Heart of Higher Education* (pp. 203–212). Springer eBooks.
- Papadopoulos, I. (2017). Intercultural Compassion in Higher Education. In *The Pedagogy of Compassion at the Heart of Higher Education* (pp. 73–84). Springer eBooks.
- Williams, J. R. (2021, November 1). *Rethinking Assessment, Equity and Academic Integrity.* Diverse: Issues in Higher Education.

Chapter 16. Facilitation Skills & Intergroup Dialogue

- Adams, M., Bell, L. A., Goodman, D. J., & Joshi, K. Y. (2016). *Teaching for Diversity and Social Justice* (4th ed.). Routledge.
- Craig, S. (2021, May 21). *When Neutrality Isn't Enough: Exploring multipartiality in the classroom.* The Georgetown Voice.
- Dessel, A., Bolen, R., & Shepardson, C. (2012). Hopes for Intergroup Dialogue: Affirmation and Allies. *Journal of Social Work Education, 48*(2), 361–367.

- Garrison, D. R., Anderson, T., & Archer, W. (2000). Critical Inquiry in a Text-Based Environment: Computer Conferencing in Higher Education. *Internet and Higher Education, 2*(2-3), 87–105.
- Lopez, G. E., & Zúñiga, X. (2010). Intergroup dialogue and democratic practice in higher education. *New Directions for Higher Education, 2010*(152), 35–42.

Chapter 17. Support Through Restorative Justice

- Ahlin, E. M., Gibbs, J. C., Kavanaugh, P. R., & Lee, J. (2016). Support for Restorative Justice in a Sample of U.S. University Students. *International Journal of Offender Therapy and Comparative Criminology, 61*(2), 229–245.
- Haines, S. (2019). *The politics of trauma : somatics, healing, and social justice.* North Atlantic Books.
- Karp, D. R. (2019). *The little book of restorative justice for colleges and universities: repairing harm and rebuilding trust in response to student misconduct* (2nd ed.). Good Books.
- Karp, D. R., & Sacks, C. (2014). Student conduct, restorative justice, and student development: findings from the STARR project: a student accountability and restorative research project. *Contemporary Justice Review, 17*(2), 154–172.
- Sopcak, P., & Hood, K. (2022). Building a Culture of Restorative Practice and Restorative Responses to Academic Misconduct. In *Academic Integrity in Canada* (Vol. 1, pp. 553–571).
- Winslade, J. (2018). Restorative Justice and Social Justice. *Journal of Critical Issues in Educational Practice, 8*(1).
- Zehr, H. (2002). *The little book of restorative justice.* Good Books.

Chapter 18. Fostering Affirming Learning Spaces

- *#HonorNativeLand.* (n.d.). U.S. Department of Arts and Culture. https://usdac.us/nativeland/
- Alicea, C. C. M., & Johnson, R. E. (2021). Creating Community Through Affinity Groups for Minority Students in Communication Sciences and Disorders. *American Journal of Speech-Language Pathology, 30*(5), 2028–2031.
- Centers for Disease Control and Prevention. (2023, April 4). *Data & statistics on autism spectrum disorder.* Centers for Disease Control and Prevention; CDC.
- Henshaw, L. A. (2022). Building Trauma-Informed Approaches in Higher Education. *Behavioral Sciences, 12*(10), 368.
- Marya, R., & Patel, R. (2021). *Inflamed: Deep Medicine and the Anatomy of Injustice* (1st ed.). Farrar, Straus and Giroux.
- Nelson, R. H. (2020). A Critique of the Neurodiversity View. *Journal of Applied Philosophy, 38*(2).

- Özlem Sensoy, & DiAngelo, R. (2014). Respect Differences? Challenging the Common Guidelines in Social Justice Education. *Democracy & Education*, 22(2), 1.
- Pour-Khorshid, F. (2018). Cultivating Sacred Spaces: A Racial Affinity Group Approach to Support Critical Educators of Color. *Teaching Education*, 29(4), 318–329.
- Spencer, S. A., Riley, A. C., & Young, S. R. (2021). Experiential education accommodations for students with disabilities in United States pharmacy schools: An exploratory study. *Currents in Pharmacy Teaching and Learning*, 13(6), 594–598.
- Tatum, B. D. (2017). *Why Are All the Black Kids Sitting Together in the Cafeteria?* Basic Books.

Chapter 19. Bias Intervention Techniques

- Ackerman-Barger, K., & Jacobs, N. N. (2020). The Microaggressions Triangle Model. *Academic Medicine*, 95(12S Addressing Harmful Bias and Eliminating Discrimination in Health Professions Learning Environments), S28–S32.
- Ackerman-Barger, K., Jacobs, N. N., Orozco, R., & London, M. (2021). Addressing Microaggressions in Academic Health: A Workshop for Inclusive Excellence. *MedEdPORTAL*, 17:11103.
- Carter, B. M., & McMillian-Bohler, J. (2020). Rewriting the Microaggression Narrative. *Nurse Educator*, 46(2), 96–100.
- Chapman, E. N., Kaatz, A., & Carnes, M. (2013). Physicians and Implicit Bias: How Doctors May Unwittingly Perpetuate Health Care Disparities. *Journal of General Internal Medicine*, 28(11), 1504–1510.
- Dyrbye, L. N., West, C. P., Sinsky, C. A., Trockel, M., Tutty, M., Satele, D., Carlasare, L., & Shanafelt, T. (2022). Physicians' Experiences With Mistreatment and Discrimination by Patients, Families, and Visitors and Association With Burnout. *JAMA Network Open*, 5(5), e2213080.
- Greenwald, A. G., McGhee, D. E., & Schwartz, J. L. K. (1998). Implicit Association Test. *PsycTESTS Dataset.*
- Hagiwara, N., Slatcher, R. B., Eggly, S., & Penner, L. A. (2016). Physician Racial Bias and Word Use during Racially Discordant Medical Interactions. *Health Communication*, 32(4), 401–408.
- Maina, I. W., Belton, T. D., Ginzberg, S., Singh, A., & Johnson, T. J. (2018). A decade of studying implicit racial/ethnic bias in healthcare providers using the implicit association test. *Social Science & Medicine*, 199(199), 219–229.
- Nakae, S., Palermo, A.-G. S., Sun, M., Roohi Byakod, & La, T. (2022). Bias Breakers: Continuous Practice for Admissions and Selection Committees. *MedEdPORTAL*, 18:11285.

- Nong, P., Raj, M., Creary, M., Kardia, S. L. R., & Platt, J. E. (2020). Patient-Reported Experiences of Discrimination in the US Health Care System. *JAMA Network Open, 3*(12), e2029650.
- Paul-Emile, K., Critchfield, J. M., Wheeler, M., de Bourmont, S., & Fernandez, A. (2020). Addressing Patient Bias Toward Health Care Workers: Recommendations for Medical Centers. *Annals of Internal Medicine, 173*(6), 468–473.
- Paul-Emile, K. (2019). How Should Organizations Support Trainees in the Face of Patient Bias? *AMA Journal of Ethics, 21*(6), E513-520.
- Sudol, N. T., Guaderrama, N. M., Honsberger, P., Weiss, J., Li, Q., & Whitcomb, E. L. (2021). Prevalence and Nature of Sexist and Racial/Ethnic Microaggressions Against Surgeons and Anesthesiologists. *JAMA Surgery, 156*(5), e210265.
- Sun, M., Oliwa, T., Peek, M. E., & Tung, E. L. (2022). Negative Patient Descriptors: Documenting Racial Bias In The Electronic Health Record. *Health Affairs, 41*(2), 203-211.
- Turner, J., Higgins, R., & Childs, E. (2021). Microaggression and Implicit Bias. *American Surgeon, 87*(11), 1727–1731.
- Vela, M. B., Erondu, A. I., Smith, N. A., Peek, M. E., Woodruff, J. N., & Chin, M. H. (2022). Eliminating explicit and implicit biases in health care: Evidence and research needs. *Annual Review of Public Health, 43*(1).

Chapter 20. "Cultural Competence" in the Curriculum

- Agner, J. (2020). Moving From Cultural Competence to Cultural Humility in Occupational Therapy: A Paradigm Shift. *American Journal of Occupational Therapy, 74*(4), 7404347010p1.
- Ambrose, A. J. H., Andaya, J. M., Yamada, S., & Maskarinec, G. G. (2014). Social justice in medical education: strengths and challenges of a student-driven social justice curriculum. *Hawai'i Journal of Medicine & Public Health, 73*(8), 244–250.
- Association of American Medical Colleges. (n.d.). *Tool for Assessing Cultural Competence Training (TACCT)*. AAMC.
- Brottman, M. R., Char, D. M., Hattori, R. A., Heeb, R., & Taff, S. D. (2019). Toward cultural competency in health care. *Academic Medicine, 95*(5), 1.
- Butler, L., Chen, A. M. H., Borja-Hart, N., Arif, S., Armbruster, A. L., Petry, N., & Riley, A. C. (2020). Assessment of a multi-institution integration of cultural competency activities. *Currents in Pharmacy Teaching and Learning, 12*(5), 517–523.
- Campinha-Bacote, J. (2002). The Process of Cultural Competence in the Delivery of Healthcare Services: A Model of Care. *Journal of Transcultural Nursing, 13*(3), 181–184.
- Clark, L., Calvillo, E., dela Cruz, F., Fongwa, M., Kools, S., Lowe, J., & Mastel-Smith, B. (2011). Cultural Competencies for Graduate Nursing Education. *Journal of Professional Nursing, 27*(3), 133–139.

- Freire, P. (2017). *Pedagogy of the Oppressed.* Penguin Books. (Original work published 1970)
- Khatri RB, Wolka E, Nigatu F, Zewdie, A., Erku DA, Endalamaw A, & Assefa, Y. (2023). People-centred primary health care: a scoping review. *BMC Primary Care, 24*(1), 236.
- Kripalani, S., Bussey-Jones, J., Katz, M. G., & Genao, I. (2006). A prescription for cultural competence in medical education. *Journal of General Internal Medicine, 21*(10), 1116–1120.
- Metzl, J. M., & Hansen, H. (2014). Structural competency: Theorizing a new medical engagement with stigma and inequality. *Social Science & Medicine, 103,* 126–133.
- Purnell, L. (2002). The Purnell Model for Cultural Competence. *Journal of Transcultural Nursing, 13*(3), 193–196.
- Rentmeester, C. A., Chapple, H. S., Haddad, A. M., & Stone, J. R. (2016). Teaching and Learning Health Justice: Best Practices and Recommendations for Innovation. *International Journal of Learning in Higher Education, 28*(3), 440–450.
- WHO. (2023). Integrated people-centred care - *GLOBAL.* www.who.int.

Chapter 21. Health Equity in Experiential Teaching

- Ahmed, S. M., Neu Young, S., DeFino, M. C., Franco, Z., & Nelson, D. A. (2017). Towards a practical model for community engagement: Advancing the art and science in academic health centers. *Journal of Clinical and Translational Science, 1*(5), 310–315.
- Ansell, MD, D. A. (2017). *The Death Gap.* University of Chicago Press.
- Cerdeña, J. P., Plaisime, M. V., & Tsai, J. (2020a). From race-based to race-conscious medicine: how anti-racist uprisings call us to act. *The Lancet, 396*(10257), 1125–1128.
- Cerdeña, J. P., Plaisime, M. V., & Tsai, J. (2020b). Race Conscious Medicine: A Reality Check [Video]. In *The Lancet.*
- Chang, A. Y., Bass, T. L., Duwell, M., Berger, J. S., Raksha Bangalore, Lee, N. S., Amdur, R. L., Andrews, M., Fahnestock, E., Kahsay, L., & Jehan El-Bayoumi. (2017). The Impact of "See the City You Serve" Field Trip: An Educational Tool for Teaching Social Determinants of Health. *Journal of Graduate Medical Education, 9*(1), 118–122.
- Roberts, D. (2012). Fatal Invention. In *The New Press* (p. 400). The New Press.
- Sabo, S., de Zapien, J., Teufel-Shone, N., Rosales, C., Bergsma, L., & Taren, D. (2015). Service Learning: A Vehicle for Building Health Equity and Eliminating Health Disparities. *American Journal of Public Health, 105*(S1), S38–S43.
- Vyas, D. A., Eisenstein, L. G., & Jones, D. S. (2020). Hidden in Plain Sight — Reconsidering the Use of Race Correction in Clinical Algorithms. *New England Journal of Medicine, 383*(9), 874–882.

Chapter 22. Case-Based Learning and Simulations

- Amutah, C., Greenidge, K., Mante, A., Munyikwa, M., Surya, S. L., Higginbotham, E., Jones, D. S., Lavizzo-Mourey, R., Roberts, D., Tsai, J., & Aysola, J. (2021). Misrepresenting Race — The Role of Medical Schools in Propagating Physician Bias. *New England Journal of Medicine, 384*(9), 872–878.
- Charon, R. (2001). Narrative medicine: a model for empathy, reflection, profession, and trust. *JAMA, 286*(15), 1897.
- Clary, K., Bennett, K., Bui, T., Tan, K., & Carter-Black, J. (2022). Simulation-Based Learning to Foster Critical Dialogues and Enhance Cultural Competency with MSW Students. *Journal of Social Work Education, 59*(4), 977–990.
- Colvin, A. D., Saleh, M., Ricks, N., & Rosa-Davila, E. (2020). Using Simulated Instruction to Prepare Students to Engage in Culturally Competent Practice. *Journal of Social Work in the Global Community, 5*(1).
- Hafferty, F. W., Gaufberg, E. H., & O'Donnell, J. F. (2015). The Role of the Hidden Curriculum in "On Doctoring" Courses. *AMA Journal of Ethics, 17*(2), 129–137.
- Kripalani, S., Bussey-Jones, J., Katz, M. G., & Genao, I. (2006). A prescription for cultural competence in medical education. *Journal of General Internal Medicine, 21*(10), 1116–1120.
- Okoro, O. N., Arya, V., Gaither, C. A., & Tarfa, A. (2021). Examining the Inclusion of Race and Ethnicity in Patient Cases. *American Journal of Pharmaceutical Education, 85*(9), 8583.
- Robertson, W. J. (2017). The Irrelevance Narrative: Queer (In)Visibility in Medical Education and Practice. *Medical Anthropology Quarterly, 31*(2), 159–176.
- Wolfe, T. (2022). *Last Summer on State Street*. HarperCollins.

Chapter 23. Decolonizing the Curriculum

- Charles, E. (2019). Decolonizing the curriculum. *Insights, 32*(1), 24.
- *Effective Teaching Is Anti-Racist Teaching | Sheridan Center | Brown University*. (n.d.). www.brown.edu.
- Hartland, J., & Larkai, E. (2020). Decolonising medical education and exploring White fragility. *BJGP Open, 4*(5), BJGPO.2020.0147.
- Kendi, I. X., & Stone, N. (2023). *How to Be a (Young) Antiracist*. Penguin.
- Levey, A. S., Coresh, J., Greene, T., Stevens, L. A., Zhang, Y. L., Hendriksen, S., Kusek, J. W., Van Lente, F., & Chronic Kidney Disease Epidemiology Collaboration. (2006). Using standardized serum creatinine values in the modification of diet in renal disease study equation for estimating glomerular filtration rate. *Medical Anthropology Quarterly, 145*(4), 247–254.
- Lokugamage, A. U., Ahillan, T., & Pathberiya, S. D. C. (2020). Decolonising ideas of healing in medical education. *Journal of Medical Ethics, 46*(4), 265–272.

- Nazar, M., Kendall, K., Day, L., & Nazar, H. (2014). Decolonising medical curricula through diversity education: Lessons from students. *Medical Teacher, 37*(4), 385–393.
- Vyas, D. A., Eisenstein, L. G., & Jones, D. S. (2020). Hidden in Plain Sight — Reconsidering the Use of Race Correction in Clinical Algorithms. *New England Journal of Medicine, 383*(9).

Chapter 24. Sustainability and Metrics for Progress

- Chisholm-Burns, M. A., Spivey, C. A., & Tipton, N. G. (2022). A diversity index to measure underrepresented minority enrollment in United States colleges and schools of pharmacy. *Currents in Pharmacy Teaching and Learning, 14*(11), 1340–1347.
- Gehlbach, H., & Brinkworth, M. E. (2011). Measure Twice, Cut down Error: A Process for Enhancing the Validity of Survey Scales. *Review of General Psychology, 15*(4), 380–387.
- Gehlbach, H., & Moulton, S. (2023, August). *Panorama Student Survey | Panorama Education.* www.panoramaed.com. https://www.panoramaed.com/panorama-student-survey
- Gomez, L. E., & Bernet, P. (2019). Diversity Improves Performance and Outcomes. *Journal of the National Medical Association, 111*(4), 383–392.
- Hagerty, B. M. K., & Patusky, K. (1995). Developing a measure of sense of belonging. *Nursing Research, 44*(1), 9–13.
- Henderson, M. C., Fancher, T. L., & Murin, S. (2023). Holistic Admissions at UC Davis—Journey Toward Equity. *Journal of the American Medical Association Network, 330*(11), 1037–1038.
- Hinton, A., & Lambert, W. M. (2022). Moving diversity, equity, and inclusion from opinion to evidence. *Cell Reports Medicine, 3*(1), 100619.
- Knekta, E., Chatzikyriakidou, K., & McCartney, M. (2020). Evaluation of a Questionnaire Measuring University Students' Sense of Belonging to and Involvement in a Biology Department. *CBE—Life Sciences Education, 19*(3), ar27, 1–14.
- Livingston, R. (2020, September 1). *How to Promote Racial Equity in the Workplace.* Harvard Business Review.
- McLaughlin, J. E., McLaughlin, G. W., McLaughlin, J. S., & White, C. Y. (2016). Using Simpson's diversity index to examine multidimensional models of diversity in health professions education. *International Journal of Medical Education, 7*, 1–5.
- Rao, K. V., Mitrzyk, B. M., Tillman, F., Liu, I., Abdul-Mutakabbir, J. C., Harvin, A., Bogucki, C., & Salsberg, E. (2023). Utilization of a "Diversity Index" to Assess Racial Diversity of US School of Pharmacy Graduates. *American Journal of Pharmaceutical Education, 87*(12), 100568.

- Rotenstein, L. S., Reede, J. Y., & Jena, A. B. (2021). Addressing Workforce Diversity — A Quality-Improvement Framework. *New England Journal of Medicine, 384*(12), 1083–1086.
- Yorke, M. (2014). The development and initial use of a survey of student "belongingness", engagement and self-confidence in UK higher education. *Assessment & Evaluation in Higher Education, 41*(1), 154–166.

Chapter 25. Continuing Professional Development

- Castillo-Montoya, M., Bolitzer, L. A., & Sotto-Santiago, S. (2023). Reimagining Faculty Development: Activating Faculty Learning for Diversity, Equity, and Inclusion. In *Higher Education: Handbook of Theory and Research* (pp. 415–481). Springer.
- Cawcutt, K. A., Erdahl, L. M., Englander, M. J., Radford, D. M., Oxentenko, A. S., Girgis, L., Migliore, L. L., Poorman, J. A., & Silver, J. K. (2019). Use of a Coordinated Social Media Strategy to Improve Dissemination of Research and Collect Solutions Related to Workforce Gender Equity. *Journal of Women's Health, 28*(6), 849–862.
- Corsino, L., & Fuller, A. T. (2021). Educating for diversity, equity, and inclusion: A review of commonly used educational approaches. *Journal of Clinical and Translational Science, 5*(1), e169.
- Costino, K. (2018). Equity-Minded Faculty Development: An Intersectional Identity-Conscious Community of Practice Model for Faculty Learning. *Metropolitan Universities, 29*(1).
- Esparza, C. J., Simon, M., Bath, E., & Ko, M. (2022). Doing the Work—or Not: The Promise and Limitations of Diversity, Equity, and Inclusion in US Medical Schools and Academic Medical Centers. *Frontiers in Public Health, 10*, 900283.
- Harte, A. (2022, April 22). *6 Strategies for Successful Diversity, Equity, and Inclusion Training*. Edutopia.
- Rodríguez, J. E., Campbell, K. M., & Pololi, L. H. (2015). Addressing disparities in academic medicine: what of the minority tax? *BMC Medical Education, 15*(1).
- Singal, J. (2023, January 17). Opinion | What if Diversity Trainings Are Doing More Harm Than Good? *The New York Times*.

Chapter 26. Organizational Culture & Inclusive Leadership

- Association of American Medical Colleges. (n.d.). *Diversity and Inclusion Toolkit Resources*. AAMC.
- Bourke, J., & Titus, A. (2020, March 6). The key to inclusive leadership. *Harvard Business Review*.
- Brown, J. (2021). *HOW TO BE AN INCLUSIVE LEADER* : your role in creating cultures of belonging where everyone can thrive. Berrett-Koehler.

- Clark, T. R. (2020). *The 4 stages of psychological safety: Defining the path to inclusion and innovation.* Berrett-Koehler Publishers, Inc.
- Relias. (2023). *2023 State of Healthcare Training and Staff Development Report.*
- Salovey, P., & Mayer, J. D. (1990). Emotional Intelligence. *Imagination, Cognition and Personality, 9*(3), 185–211.
- Shore, L. M., Randel, A. E., Chung, B. G., Dean, M. A., Holcombe Ehrhart, K., & Singh, G. (2011). Inclusion and Diversity in Work Groups: A Review and Model for Future Research. *Journal of Management, 37*(4), 1262–1289.
- Slootman, M. (2022). Affinity networks as diversity instruments. Three sociological dilemmas. *Scandinavian Journal of Management, 38*(3), 101217.
- Tabak, L. (2023). *Fiscal Years 2023-2027 NIH-Wide Strategic Plan for DEIA i.*
- The Joint Commission. (2010). *A Roadmap for Hospitals Advancing Effective Communication, Cultural Competence, and Patient-and Family-Centered Care Quality Safety Equity.*
- Winters, M.-F. (2017). *We can't talk about that at work! how to talk about race, religion, politics, and other polarizing topics.* Berrett-Koehler Publishers, Inc.
- Zheng, W., Kim, J., Kark, R., & Mascolo, L. (2023, September 27). *What Makes an Inclusive Leader?* Harvard Business Review.

Acknowledgments

First and foremost, I must express my boundless gratitude to my Creator, the Ever-Magnificent and Ever-Merciful, for granting me the opportunity, courage, and energy to complete this book. Any benefit gained from this work is from Him, while any mistakes are my own.

To my beloved husband, Mustafa, and my two wonderful children—your unwavering support and love have been my constant source of motivation and joy. Thank you to my dear mother, father, and brothers—your love, sacrifices, and belief in me have been the foundation of my strength and perseverance.

I am immensely grateful to all my formal and informal teachers who have provided me with the encouragement and wisdom to strive for excellence and become a better version of myself. To my community of friends who are like family, from The Gambia to Chicago and beyond: the light of your *suhba* (companionship) continues to be a guiding force in my life.

To those who have walked alongside me in my professional development, thank you for amplifying my voice even when it was shaky—your support has not gone unnoticed. To all my former students and residents who have shared your hearts with me over the years, I will always treasure your stories. They have profoundly shaped my embodied approach to cultivating equity and inclusion.

I extend my deepest gratitude to the many individuals who believed in my message and for your tireless guidance in bringing this book to life, despite the many unforseen challenges. My heartfelt gratitude goes to Nermin Moufti for applying her brilliant creative design talent to the cover, embodying the essence of this work.

I also wish to express my sincere appreciation to Shazia Pappa for her expertise in crafting impactful figures that elevate the content. A heartfelt thank you to my peer reviewers: Brooke Griffin, Kruti Parikh Shah, Melisa Alabsy, Saira Doja, Brianna Spurlock, Simi Burn, and Titilola Afolabi—your feedback and encouragement have been instrumental in steering this book to the finish line. I hope the final version makes you proud.

I also want to acknowledge all the fierce advocates in my circle who continue to dedicate their efforts to the pursuit of equity, inclusion, and social justice in healthcare and higher education. Your bravery continues to motivate me. I deeply appreciate our reciprocal mentorship and the space you hold for me to share my setbacks, challenges, joy, and wins.

Health Equity Pedagogical Resources

Scan this code to access exclusive health equity pedagogical resources and tools available through www.equitymindedcollective.com.

www.ingramcontent.com/pod-product-compliance
Lightning Source LLC
Chambersburg PA
CBHW020532030426
42337CB00013B/819